Orthopaedics for Undergraduates

BY
C. J. E. MONK

M.B., B.Ch. (Witwatersrand), M.Ch.Orth. (Liverpool),
F.R.C.S. (Edin), F.R.C.S. (Eng.),
Consultant Orthopaedic Surgeon,
Liverpool Area Health Authority

OXFORD UNIVERSITY PRESS
1976

Oxford University Press, Ely House, London W.1

GLASGOW NEW YORK TORONTO MELBOURNE WELLINGTON
CAPE TOWN IBADAN NAIROBI DAR ES SALAAM LUSAKA ADDIS ABABA
DELHI BOMBAY CALCUTTA MADRAS KARACHI LAHORE DACCA
KUALA LUMPUR SINGAPORE HONG KONG TOKYO

ISBN 0 19 265206 0

© Oxford University Press 1976

All rights reserved. No part of this publication may be reproduced, stored in a retrieval system, or transmitted, in any form or by any means, electronic, mechanical, photocopying, recording or otherwise, without the prior permission of Oxford University Press

This book is sold subject to the condition that it shall not, by way of trade or otherwise, be lent, re-sold, hired out, or otherwise circulated without the publisher's prior consent in any form of binding or cover other than that in which it is published and without a similar condition including this condition being imposed on the subsequent purchaser.

Drawings by David Woodroffe

Printed in Great Britain by J. W. Arrowsmith Ltd., Bristol

Preface

I have produced this book in order to give the undergraduate student an idea of the scope of orthopaedics and traumatology. It is intended to be used in conjunction with lectures, demonstrations, ward rounds, and clinics.

Emphasis is placed on the clinical presentation of the conditions described. The principles of treatment are described but the finer details of operative technique are omitted as I feel that these are more the concern of the postgraduate student.

Although the majority of the views given in the book conform to traditional Liverpool teaching, it must be emphasized that the philosophy of treatment is that of the author and that the student may encounter different methods of treatment in other hospitals.

At the end of most of the chapters the student will find a list of references for further reading. These references will also introduce the student to the use of the Periodicals section of the library if he is not already acquainted with it, and, I hope, whet his appetite for exploring in some detail any aspect of the subject which appeals to him.

I would like to acknowledge the help and encouragement given to me by Professor Roaf, and would like to thank all my colleagues who have allowed me access to clinical photographs and radiographs used as a basis for the line diagrams.

Liverpool, 1975 C. J. E. M.

Contents

PART I
GENERAL CONDITIONS OF THE MUSCULO-SKELETAL SYSTEM

1.	Introduction to terminology	3
2.	Principles of clinical assessment	6
3.	Fractures and dislocations	15
4.	The management of the severely injured patient	21
5.	Conditions affecting peripheral nerves	25
6.	Rheumatoid disease	33
7.	Cerebral palsy and poliomyelitis	36
8.	Infections of bone	41
9.	Infections of joints	47
10.	Degenerative arthrosis	51
11.	Generalized conditions of bone	55
12.	Conditions of tendons and tendon sheaths	67
13.	Bone and soft-tissue tumours	72
14.	Other conditions of joints	83

PART II
REGIONAL CONDITIONS

15.	The neck	91
16.	The thoracic spine	101
17.	The lumbar spine	105
18.	The pelvis and sacrum	116
19.	The shoulder region	121
20.	The arm	129
21.	The elbow region	131

22.	The forearm	142
23.	The wrist region	146
24.	The hand and fingers	155
25.	The hip region	166
26.	The thigh	180
27.	The knee region	184
28.	The leg	196
29.	The ankle region	201
30.	The foot and toes	209
Index		219

PART I
General conditions of the musculo-skeletal system

1 Introduction to terminology

We find that the main difficulty experienced by students starting their orthopaedic attachment is that of understanding the terms and expressions used. For this reason I start with a short introduction to terminology. The following terms will crop up repeatedly during your attachment to the orthopaedic firms.

Deformity
A deformity is an abnormality in shape which is visible.

Congenital
Congenital means present at birth. It should be realized that an abnormality may be present at birth (i.e. congenital) but that its effects on appearance may not be apparent until the child has grown to some extent, i.e. the deformity is not congenital but the cause is.

Valgus and varus
These terms are used mainly to describe deformities. A deformity of a bone or joint which causes angulation of the limb distal to the point of deformity away from the midline is called a valgus deformity. A deformity which causes the

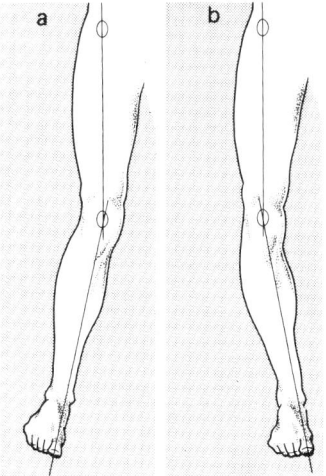

FIG. 1.1. (a) Valgus deformity of knee (genu valgum).
(b) Varus deformity of knee (genu varum).

limb distal to it to be angled towards the midline is a varus deformity. It is important to place the limb proximal to the deformity in its anatomical position before commenting on the type of deformity: e.g., a bow-leg deformity at the knee will be found to be a varus deformity at the knee, if this is done, because the tibia is angled medially on the femur. Similarly, a knock-knee deformity is a valgus deformity at the knee (Fig. 1.1).

Remember that the definition of valgus and varus depends on the angulation of the limb *distal* to the deformity.

In orthopaedics we tend to use the Latin names for joints, e.g. genu varum and valgum (knee), cubitus varus and valgus (elbow), and coxa vara and valga (hip region).

Parts of the bone

You are probably well aware of the parts of an adult bone, e.g. shaft, head, tuberosity, and articular surface. Students, however, appear to have some difficulty with the nomenclature of the parts of a developing bone. This is best resolved by a rapid survey of bone development.

In utero, foetal bones are mainly laid down as a cartilage template (Fig. 1.2(a)). Ossification starts in the centre of the bone ('primary' area of ossification) and progresses towards either end so that by birth most of what is later to become the shaft of the bone is ossified but the ends are still cartilaginous (Fig. 1.2(b)). During the first few years of life 'secondary' centres of ossification appear in the cartilaginous ends of the bones and they become changed to bone (Fig. 1.2.(c)). A thin area of cartilage remains unossified between the primary and secondary areas of ossification. If we refer to this unossified area of cartilage as 'physis' (plural: physes) we can readily understand the terms applied to the developing bone (Fig. 1.2(d)).
1. The area between the physes is the diaphysis.
2. The areas beyond the physes are the epiphyses.

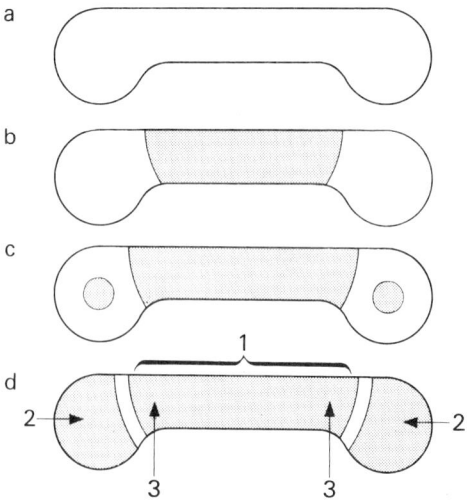

FIG. 1.2. Diagrams of developing bone (see text).

3. The area of diaphysis alongside the physis is the metaphysis.
When growth of the bone is complete these physes become ossified and the adult terminology (head, shaft, etc.) is used.

The subject is, unfortunately, slightly complicated because the term 'physis' is not used for the unossified area between metaphysis and epiphysis but instead this is referred to (incorrectly) as the epiphyseal cartilage, epiphyseal plate, or epiphyseal line.

The reason for explaining these terms in some detail is that many of the orthopaedic conditions encountered during the growing period affect specifically one part of the developing bone, e.g. osteomyelitis which affects the metaphysis, or osteochondritis which usually affects the epiphysis.

Fractures

A fracture is a break in the continuity of a bone. Even a crack in a trabeculum of the marrow space constitutes a fracture.

There are many types of fractures with terms to describe them, thus it is possible to assemble a 'catalogue' of fractures. To be of use a classification must help in the understanding of a subject or divide up conditions with regard to cause, treatment, or prognosis. We have found that there is only one useful classification of fractures.

Such a classification is into (1) simple (or closed) fractures and (2) compound (or open) fractures.

Simple fractures
The term 'simple' means that the fracture has no communication to the exterior, i.e. that the skin or mucous membrane overlying the bone is still intact and so is acting as a barrier to infecting organisms.

Compound fractures
The term 'compound' means that the fracture is open to the external environment. This means that the skin or mucous membrane (in the case of the mandible for example) is not intact and infection of the fracture site is likely. The terms 'open' and 'closed' are synonymous respectively with compound and simple.

Orthopaedics

The term 'orthopaedics' was applied to the study of the correction of deformities in children which in the 1800s constituted the bulk of the work of orthopaedic surgeons. The actual derivation is *ortho* (straight) and *paedeia* (the rearing of children).

2 Principles of clinical assessment

HISTORY

The symptoms which cause the patient to seek advice from an orthopaedic surgeon usually fall into three main groups:
(1) pain felt in the neck, back, pelvis, or limbs;
(2) awareness of abnormal appearance due to swelling, wasting, or deformity in one or more parts of the body;
(3) abnormality of the range of movement of a joint or joints (usually a decrease in the range).

Pain

It is important to determine the following points about pain:
(1) the site and radiation;
(2) the length of time for which the patient has had the pain and whether it varies in intensity;
(3) any possible original causation, e.g. accidents;
(4) factors which aggravate it;
(5) factors which relieve it;
(6) severity of pain—particularly whether it interferes with sleep.

In orthopaedics it is especially important—and often difficult—to estimate the severity of the pain as compared with the severity of the patient's reaction to the pain.

Referred pain

Pain arising in a lesion may be felt not at the lesion but in another region of the body supplied by the same spinal segment(s). This phenomenon is called 'referred pain' and is very common in orthopaedics. Examples are a degenerative hip causing pain felt on the inner side of the knee and degenerative posterior joints in the lower lumbar spine causing pain down the back of the thigh and leg. The relationship can often be proved by moving the affected area and thereby causing or increasing the pain which is felt in the area of 'referral'.

Swelling, wasting, or deformity

Here again the length of time for which the patient has been aware of the abnormality and any possible cause must be ascertained. It should be asked whether a swelling varies in size and whether it is painful. Progression of a deformity should be noted.

Changes in range of movement of joints

A diminution in joint movement range in some joints is quickly noticed by the patient, e.g. the finger joints, the knee, and the elbow. Other joints, e.g. the hip, may become almost completely stiff before the patient is aware of any change. This is usually because movement of other joints—for example the lumbar spine joints in the case of the hip—can substitute for a stiff joint and mask its lack of movement.

CLINICAL EXAMINATION

In assessing most orthopaedic complaints it is necessary to examine the patient standing, walking, and lying down. Examination should include full assessment of the limb, the contralateral limb for comparison and the relevant area of the spine. Hilton's ancient dictum that 'pain in an area is due to a lesion in that area or a lesion affecting the nerves supplying that area', is worth remembering. Other structures innervated from the same segment of the spine should also be examined.

General examination of joints

There are five manoeuvres necessary in the examination of any joint and until they have been carried out examination of the joint is not complete. This routine is based on that popularized by A. G. Apley, F.R.C.S. of Pyrford. The following procedures should be carried out on the joint:
 (1) look at;
 (2) feel;
 (3) move;
 (4) strain; and
 (5) X-ray.
1. *Looking*. The following should be noticed:
 (a) Position of the joint (and limb) at rest, e.g. painful hip is usually held flexed.
 (b) Swellings or abnormalities in contour, e.g. a synovial effusion causes filling out of the normal concavity medial to the patella.
 (c) Old scars or sinuses.
 (d) Deformities.
 (e) Skin—texture, colour, absence of hairs.
 (f) Muscle wasting.
2. *Feeling*. The following are usually palpable:
 (a) Increased temperature.
 (b) Points of tenderness.
 (c) Small swellings.
 (d) Thickening of the synovium.
 (e) Crepitus.
3. *Moving*. The patient is first asked to move the joint actively. The range of active movement is then compared with the range when the joint is moved by the examiner. The starting and finishing point of the range should be noted. In tears of the menisci, for example, the last few degrees of extension of the knee may be lost.
4. *Straining*. The ligaments of the joint are subjected to moderate strain. This will cause discomfort in recently damaged ligaments and an increased range of movement in torn or stretched ligaments.
5. *X-ray*. Two views of a joint (an antero-posterior and a lateral) are routinely

taken except in the hands and feet where the lateral view is complicated by superimposition of shadows. The outline of the articular surfaces, the depth of the 'joint space' (the area between the bones which contains the layers of articular cartilage), and the presence of osteophytes and loose bodies are noted.

Examination of individual joints

The cervical spine
The joints of the cervical spine are best examined from behind the patient. The patient is asked to flex and extend the neck, then to laterally rotate the head until the nose takes up a position vertically over the shoulder, and finally to laterally flex the neck to each side so that the ear approaches the shoulder on the same side.

These movements are repeated rapidly and the patient asked if there is any discomfort felt in the neck or upper limbs. Pain or paraesthesia felt in the upper limbs implies that the source of the patient's symptoms lies in the neck —either a 'trigger' lesion causing referred pain, or a lesion pressing on the cervical roots or nerves.

The shoulder joint
Like the cervical spine, the shoulders are best examined from behind the patient. A dislocation of the shoulder is much more obvious if the patient is seen from behind: the normal smooth curve of the deltoid is replaced by a 'squaring off' of the contour due to the relative prominence of the acromion.

It is customary to examine three ranges of movement in the shoulder: abduction; external rotation; and internal rotation.

Abduction. This movement takes place at two different sites: first at the gleno-humeral joint (the shoulder joint proper); and secondly at the interface between the scapula and the chest wall ('scapulo-thoracic region'). It is important to note how much movement takes place at each site. With the arm hanging at the side, palm facing outwards, the patient is asked to elevate the limb in the coronal plane. In a normal shoulder approximately the first 90° of movement occurs at the gleno-humeral joint and the second 90° at the scapulo-thoracic. It is advisable to palpate the scapula during this manoeuvre as it is sometimes difficult to see its range of movement.

Rotational movement. The shoulder is abducted 90° and the elbow flexed 90°. Neutral rotation is taken as the point at which the forearm is horizontal. The normal shoulder can be externally rotated 90° (i.e. ending up with the forearm vertical) and internally rotated 80° from this position. It is important to note the presence of pain or discomfort on these movements.

If abduction to 90° is not possible the rotation ranges are tested with the arm at the side. It is more difficult to estimate internal rotation in this position.

The elbow joint
The range of flexion should be tested with the forearm supinated (palm-up). The range of pronation and supination should be tested with the elbow flexed at 90°. This avoids the danger of including some degree of shoulder rotation in the pronation and supination movement which normally occurs at the superior and inferior radio-ulnar joints only.

Principles of clinical assessment

The wrist joint
It is important to palpate the range of movement of the proximal row of carpal bones in the palmar flexion and dorsiflexion range. This is because an increased range of movement in the intercarpal and carpo-metacarpal joints develops in some cases as stiffening of the wrist (radio-carpal joint). Radial and ulnar deviation are also measured.

The thumb
The confusion which usually surrounds naming the movements of the thumb can be resolved by noting that the thumb lies at rest rotated 90° along its long axis when compared to the fingers. Flexion therefore brings the distal phalanx across the palm and abduction brings it away from the index finger metacarpal in a plane at right angles to the plane of the palm.

The lumbar spine
Flexion of the lumbar spine is tested by asking the patient to touch his or her toes and then noting how much of the movement is actually due to bending of the lumbar spine. People with supple hips, e.g. ballet dancers, can touch their toes without flexing the lumbar spine at all.

Lateral flexion and rotation are also measured, the latter by asking the patient to fold his arms across his chest and then swing to the left and right.

As in the case of the cervical spine, it is important to note any discomfort felt in the lower limbs during movements of the lumbar spine.

The hip joints
Like the shoulder joint, the hip is a ball and socket joint and normally we test specific ranges of movement: flexion; abduction; adduction; and medial and lateral rotation.

The diseased hip may develop contractures and it is important to realize that these contractures may be masked by compensatory positions of other joints. The classical example of this is the flexion contracture of the hip joint. As the contracture develops the patient adapts for it—usually unconsciously—by tilting the pelvis forward. This is achieved by increasing the lordosis of the lumbar spine. If such a patient is laid supine and the pelvis tilted back to its normal position the flexion deformity of the suspect hip becomes obvious. The usual method of undoing the tilt is by hyperflexing the sound hip until the lumbar spine straightens out. This manoeuvre is referred to as Thomas' hip flexion test (Fig. 2.1).

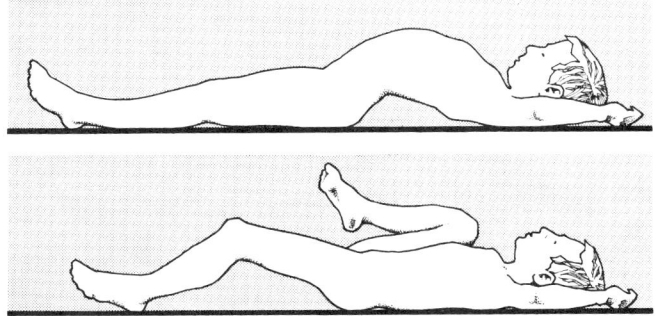

FIG. 2.1. Thomas' hip flexion test.

10 Orthopaedics for Undergraduates

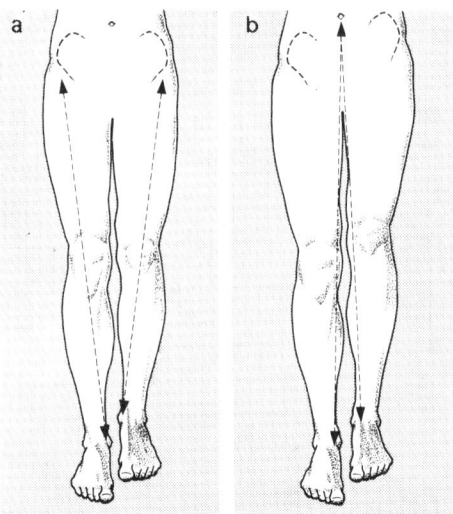

FIG. 2.2. (a) True shortening of the left lower limb.
(b) Apparent shortening of the left lower limb.

Abduction and adduction. When measuring these ranges, the examiner should keep one hand on the contralateral anterior superior iliac spine, as again contractures may be masked by movement of the pelvis. The patient may mask an adduction contracture of the hip by lying with his pelvis tilted as seen from the front. If the true lengths of his lower limbs are the same, this tilt will be demonstrated by measuring the lengths of the limbs from a central point, e.g. the umbilicus. The limb on the side of the adducted hip will be apparently shorter. These measurements of the limbs relative to a single fixed point are referred to as the 'apparent lengths' of the limbs (Fig. 2.2).

Rotational movement. In the routine examination of the hip internal and external rotation ranges are tested with the hip and knee flexed 90°. In some special cases, e.g. assessment of anteversion of the femoral neck in children, it is better to test rotation with the hip extended. Whichever method is used it must be adhered to each time the patient is examined as the ranges differ in the two positions.

Trendelenberg sign. In a patient with normal hips, when weight is taken on one leg, the pelvis on the non-weight-bearing side rises slightly. This is due to the abductors (mainly the gluteus medius) on the weight-bearing side pulling the iliac crest down towards the greater trochanter. The fulcrum for this movement is the head of the femur and the levers are the ilium and the neck of the femur. If any of these are damaged, for instance in weakness of the glutei, degenerative arthritis of the hip or injuries of the neck of the femur, this action does not occur and the pelvis on the non-weight-bearing side dips down. This constitutes a positive Trendelenberg test (Fig. 2.3).

Principles of clinical assessment 11

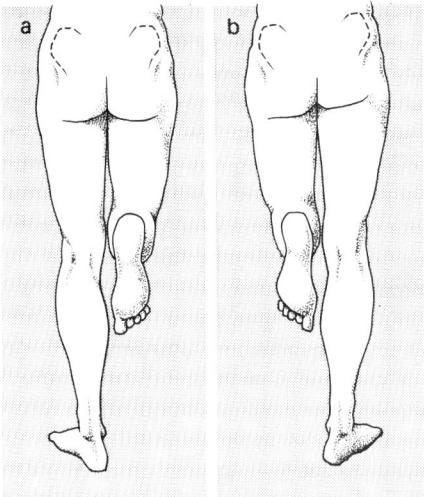

FIG. 2.3. Trendelenberg's test. (a) Negative. (b) Positive.

In walking, the patient with a positive Trendelenberg sign adapts for the dipping of the pelvis when the suspect hip is weight-bearing by leaning over the same side and so raising the pelvis on the sound side in order to allow the leg to swing through without the foot scraping along the ground. This gives rise to the characteristic Trendelenberg lurch on walking. If both hips are affected the patient lurches to either side as he walks—the 'rolling sailor gait'.

The knee joint

Range. Normally the knee joint has a range of flexion of approximately 0–150°. It is important to check this range carefully. Lack of a few degrees of extension, especially if the normal 'lock-home' feeling is replaced by a 'springy' or 'rubbery' block, may be the only sign of a damaged meniscus. Slight hyperflexion and hyperextension strain should be applied and particular note made of the site of any discomfort felt by the patient. This may be of great help in deciding which meniscus is damaged.

Synovial effusions. Effusions into the synovial cavity are common and three stages or degrees of severity are described.

First degree: Loss of the normal concavity medial to the patella.
Second degree: There is sufficient fluid present to 'float' the patella off the underlying femur, especially if the suprapatellar pouch is compressed. This permits the 'ballotting' of the patella against the femur—the so called 'patella tap'.
Third degree: A tense effusion preventing full extension of the knee.

Ligaments. The medial and lateral ligaments are tested by valgus and varus straining. The cruciate ligaments are tested by pulling the tibia forward and pushing it backward under the femur with the knee flexed 90° (the draw sign). The patient lies supine, completely relaxed, and the examiner anchors the patient's foot by sitting on it (gently).

Menisci. Tenderness over the relevant joint line is the most dependable sign of a damaged meniscus. Occasionally a loose tag of cartilage becomes folded over the remainder of the meniscus and is palpable over the joint line.

McMurray's test. Several versions of this test for torn menisci are practised. The one which we recommend is as follows.

The patient lies supine and completely relaxed. Relaxation of the hamstrings may be enhanced by getting the patient to hold his thigh. The examiner holds the suspect knee and the foot of the same limb. With his fingers or thumb over the joint line of the knee the examiner flexes the knee and hip to 90°. With the foot externally rotated and the patient fully relaxed the leg is now circumducted through circles of varying radii. A positive test consists of feeling a click over the suspect meniscus—this may be painful.

If no click is obtained, the procedure is repeated with the foot internally rotated. At the end of circumduction in each case the knee is extended with the foot held either internally or externally rotated and this occasionally produces a click. The click is produced by the damaged meniscus interfering with the knee movement.

It must be emphasized that all these tests may be negative with some types of meniscus tears.

The patella compression test. The patient is asked to lie flat and relax the quadriceps muscle. The examiner then presses the patella against the femur and the patient is asked to contract the quadriceps. A positive result (as seen in chondromalacia patellae) consists of discomfort felt to a greater extent on the suspect than on the contralateral side.

The ankle joint
This is a simple hinge joint well protected by ligaments and tendons.

Range of movement. The normal adult ankle has a range of dorsiflexion of approximately 0–30° and a plantar flexion range of approximately 0–40°. This range is sometimes difficult to measure but a good idea of the range may be obtained from watching the os calcis during its movement or by asking the patient to stand with his foot flat on the floor and then flex his leg forwards and backwards as far as he can without lifting his forefoot or heel off the ground.

In cases of torn medial or lateral ligaments of the ankle, spasm of the peronei or posterior tibial muscle groups may mask the instability of the joint. It can, however, be demonstrated by anaesthetizing the patient and taking antero-posterior radiographs with the ankle strained alternately into valgus and varus.

The sub-talar and mid-tarsal joints
Inversion and eversion of the foot takes place at these joints and students sometimes experience some difficulty in deciding how much of the movement is occurring at each joint. This can be resolved by holding the os calcis in one hand and the forefoot in the other and moving the forefoot and heel as a single unit in the first instance. Then by holding the os calcis immobile with one hand and moving the forefoot with the other, the amount of midtarsal movement can be estimated. The patient, of course, lies supine and relaxed during this manoeuvre.

Principles of clinical assessment 13

Metatarso-phalangeal joints
When a person stands, the metatarsal bones of the foot incline downwards and forwards from the tarsal region. This means that the physiological range of the metatarso-phalangeal (m.p.) joints must be mainly in the dorsiflexion range. The normal range of m.p. joint movement in the big toe is dorsiflexion 0–90° and plantar flexion 0–0° when measured from the plane of the metatarsals.

Examination of bones
The same manoeuvres are carried out as in the examination of joints—indeed the examination of a particular bone is incomplete unless the joints in which it takes part are also examined.

Examination of nerves
When asked to examine a particular nerve, students usually start with its sensory area of supply. It is, in fact, often easier and more revealing to test its motor function and power. Reflex activity as seen in tendon jerks is more often used as an assessment of spinal root abnormalities than peripheral nerve lesions as such.

Examination of deformities
Having noted the degree of the deformity it is very important to assess whether any correction can be obtained by moving the affected joint or bone. A mobile deformity is usually easier to treat than a fixed one.

Gait
If the patient is suffering from any condition which involves the lower limbs it is essential to examine his or her gait. This will give a good indication of the cause and severity of the disability and hence the need for treatment or other social or domestic arrangements.

Special types of gait
1. *Hemiplegic gait.* The patient walks with the upper limb on the affected side flexed at the elbow and wrist. The lower limb is stiff and the patient allows for the loss of knee flexion by circumducting the limb outwards. Some equinus is present at the ankle. This gait is seen in patients suffering from cerebral palsy and following cerebrovascular accidents.
2. *'Scissor gait'.* Also common in patients with cerebral palsy. Overactivity of the thigh adductors causes the patient to walk with the thighs tightly held together. In addition to the scissor gait these patients may also suffer from overactivity of knee flexors and calf muscles which cause them to walk with the knee flexed and the ankles plantar flexed—the heels are clear of the ground and the patient walks on the balls of his feet.
3. *Athetoid gait.* This is characterized by purposeless uncontrolled movement, often with loss of co-ordination.
4. *Drop-foot gait.* Seen most commonly in polio: a high-stepping gait, the foot tending to dangle in equinus when off the ground.
5. *Trendelenberg gait.* A lurch to the weight-bearing side (see p. 11).
6. *Antalgic gait.* This literally means an anti-pain gait and is usually characterized by the patient 'hurrying off' one lower limb and spending an appreciably greater part of the walking cycle on the other. It is caused by pain on weight-

bearing and seen commonly in osteoarthritis of the hip or knee in adults and painful hip and foot condition in children.

It is as well to remember the old adage that the commonest causes of limps in children are nails in the shoe and wearing shoes which are too small.

RECOMMENDATIONS FOR FURTHER READING

McMurray, T. P. (1949) General examination of the knee. In *A Practice of Orthopaedic Surgery*, p. 51, Edward Arnold, London.

Rang, M. (1966) Trendelenberg test—original description. In *Anthology of Orthopaedics*, pp. 139–43, E. & S. Livingstone, Edinburgh.

General reference

Gillis, L. (1969) *Diagnosis in Orthopaedics*, Butterworths, London.

3 Fractures and dislocations

FRACTURES

Definition

A fracture is a break in the continuity of a bone. It is important to realize that any break, even of one cortex, constitutes a fracture.

Classification

Fractures may be simple or compound.

Simple fracture
This implies that there is no contact with the external environment, i.e. the skin or mucous membrane overlying the bone is intact.

Compound fracture
This implies that there is direct contact between the fracture and the external environment, e.g. a fracture of the tibia with a laceration of the overlying skin, or a fracture of the mandible with laceration of the overlying mucous membrane.

This is a useful classification because compound fractures are likely to become infected and simple fractures are not.

Other descriptive terms for fractures
Several terms are used to describe fractures:
1. *Comminuted.* There are more than two fragments present.
2. *Complicated.* There is some important structure, a nerve, artery, or viscus, involved in the fracture.
3. *Pathological.* The fracture has occurred in abnormal bone.
4. *Stress.* The fracture has resulted from repeated application of minor force rather than one large force.
5. *Greenstick.* Only one cortex of the bone as seen on X-ray is fractured.

It is important to appreciate that these are descriptive terms. The only classification of fractures is into simple (closed) and compound (open) fractures.

Symptoms

Virtually all fractures are painful and caused by the application of force. The amount of force may be small, especially in pathological fracture. Often a patient will give a history of hearing a crack or of feeling the bone give way

Signs

There are three classical signs of a fracture but they may not all be present.
1. The limb looks deformed. The deformity is due to angulation,

16 *Orthopaedics for Undergraduates*

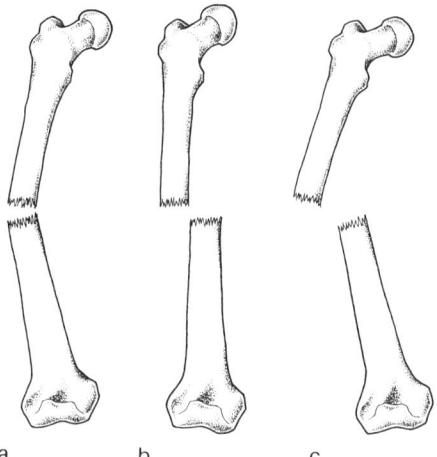

FIG. 3.1. Fracture deformity due to: (a) angulation; (b) displacement; (c) angulation and displacement.

displacement, or angulation and displacement combined (Fig. 3.1).
2. The fracture site is tender to palpation.
3. There is unnatural mobility at the fracture site.

Treatment of simple fractures

There are three principles of treatment of a simple fracture: reduction, immobilization, and protection.

The fragments are replaced in their proper alignment. This implies that the angulation or displacement is *reduced*. In everyday parlance this has been shortened to the expression 'the fracture is reduced'. Reduction, of course, is necessary only in displaced or angulated fractures.

The bone is held in the realigned position until the processes of healing have caused the fragments to stick together again or 'unite'. This holding of the bone fragments is referred to as *immobilization*.

After union, the bone takes some time to regain its pre-fracture strength and so the fracture is *protected* until this strengthening is complete. When this has occurred the fracture is referred to as 'consolidated'.

In summary, therefore, the treatment of a simple fracture consists of:
(1) reduction;
(2) immobilization until united; and
(3) protection until consolidated.

Methods of reduction of fractures
Manipulation. The vast majority of fractures can be reduced by manipulation of the bone fragments with the patient anaesthetized. Occasionally, however, reduction is not achieved because of soft tissue interposition or because it is impossible to obtain a sufficient hold on one or other fragments. It may be necessary therefore to operate on the fracture in order to reduce it. This is referred to as open reduction.

Open reduction. In this method the surgeon exposes the bone-ends and realigns them. This obviously converts a simple fracture to a compound fracture with the danger of infection. If it is known that a certain fracture will require internal fixation (see below), the reduction is usually carried out at the time of fixation and is therefore an open reduction.

Open reduction of a fracture is indicated when closed reduction is impossible or unsatisfactory.

Methods of immobilization or fixation of fractures
External fixation. Most fractures of limbs can be satisfactorily fixed by external means, of which there are three main types.
1. Splints—usually made of metal and held on by bandages.
2. Plaster of Paris casts.
3. Traction—applying a pulling force along the line of a limb places the muscles surrounding the fracture under tension and this holds the fracture reduced. This principle is used in the Thomas splint.

Internal fixation. This is used where external fixation is unsuitable, either because it does not hold the fracture satisfactorily, or because it constitutes a risk to the patient, e.g. immobilizing the hip in a plaster cast in an old person with a fracture of the neck of the femur will probably lead to the development of hypostatic pneumonia and pressure sores.

The devices used for internal fixation of the fractures are three main types.
1. Intramedullary rods and nails used for fractures of long bones.
2. Plates held on with screws.
3. Screws to hold small fragments in place or to hold against redisplacement when the overall immobilization is achieved by a plaster cast.

Some fractures, e.g. in the trochanteric area of the femur, are held by a combination of an intramedullary pin in the neck attached to a plate on the upper shaft.

Internal fixation, then, is indicated when external fixation is impossible or unsatisfactory.

Assessment of union
Union is a clinical phenomenon. A fracture is said to be united when the bone moves as a single unit and is not tender to moderate stressing. The assessment of union is impossible if internal fixation has been used. The presence of callus on the radiograph is good corroborative evidence of union but does not, on its own, indicate it.

Methods of protection of fractures
Once a fracture has united, treatment of the joints in the vicinity is started in order to restore their range of movement. The fracture must be protected, however, until it has consolidated (particularly if it is in a weight-bearing bone). This protection is afforded by:
1. Crutches—the weight is taken on the upper limbs either totally or in part.
2. Splints—which protect the fracture from undue strain.
3. Calipers—a system of longitudinal iron supports either to prevent bending strains or to take the body weight off the fractured lower limb (Fig. 3.2).

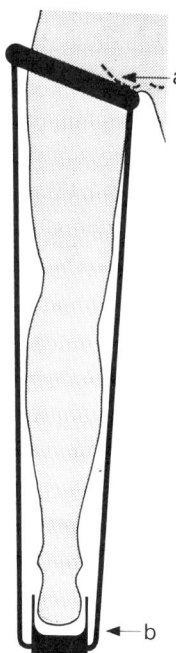

FIG. 3.2. Principle of the weight-relieving caliper. (a) The body weight is taken on the ischial tuberosity. (b) The patient's heel is lifted off the heel of the shoe.

Treatment of compound fractures

Because of the danger of infection, compound fractures are considered to be surgical emergencies. The first aim of treatment is to convert them to simple fractures by closing any passage to the exterior. Thereafter the treatment follows the same principles as for simple fractures except that the implanting of any foreign metal to hold the fragments in position should be delayed until one is satisfied that there is no infection present.

Physiological repair

Stage of haematoma formation

Following the injury the broken ends of the bone are surrounded by damaged muscles and fascia and are lying in a pool of blood. The periosteum has been stripped from the underlying bone for some distance on either side of the fracture. The haematoma clots.

Stage of proliferation

The haematoma acts as a bridge along which cells grow. Cellular proliferation from the periosteum and the endosteum now starts and the whole fracture area becomes cellular. The haematoma is gradually absorbed.

Stage of callus formation

The proliferating cells lay down intercellular substance which becomes calcified and then organized into woven bone. At this stage clinical union is noted and this 'callus' is visible on radiographs. The mass of callus is often palpable as a hard swelling at the fracture site (Latin *callus* = hard).

Stage of lamellar bone formation

The woven bone of the callus is gradually replaced by lamellar bone, i.e. bone laid down in Haversian systems. The strength of the repair is increased.

Stage of remodelling

Over the succeeding months and years the fracture callus is remodelled by the combined action of osteoblasts and osteoclasts.

Complications

You will remember that a fracture is defined as being 'complicated' if there is damage to another major structure, e.g. vessel, nerve, or viscus (p. 15). In addition to this type of complication we must consider two other types of complications, namely complications of the injury itself and complications of the healing process.

Complications of the injury

1. *Haemorrhage.* Bleeding from fractured bones and surrounding veins and arteries may be considerable. It is especially important to consider bleeding in

case of bones situated deeply in the body, e.g. the lumbar spine and pelvis, because the patient may lose 2 litres or more of blood into the loose retroperitoneal tissues without there being any overt sign of blood loss until the onset of shock.

2. *Sepsis.* This is particularly seen in compound fractures and may lead to chronic osteomyelitis. Union may be delayed.

Complications of fracture healing

1. *Delayed union.* This is said to have occurred when a fracture has not united in a reasonable time. A reasonable time is defined as 25 per cent longer than the average time taken for this type of fracture to unite. The main causes of delayed union are:
   (a) inadequate immobilization;
   (b) interposition of soft tissues;
   (c) sepsis; or
   (d) poor blood-supply of fracture site.

The last is seen in some fractures of the tibia: at three months the bone-ends show very little change from their appearance at the time of the accident.

2. *Non-union.* The actual point in time when one stops referring to delayed union and calls the phenomenon 'non-union' is a debatable one but most authorities consider one year a reasonable period.

3. *Mal-union.* This term is used when a fracture has united out of alignment. It may or may not be significant; some displacement of fractures of the femoral shaft is acceptable, but angulation in fractures of the radius or ulna is not acceptable because of interference with pronation and supination.

DISLOCATIONS AND SUBLUXATIONS

Definitions

A dislocation is a displacement of the articular surfaces of the bones forming a joint to such an extent that there is no contact between them (the old name for dislocation was 'luxation').

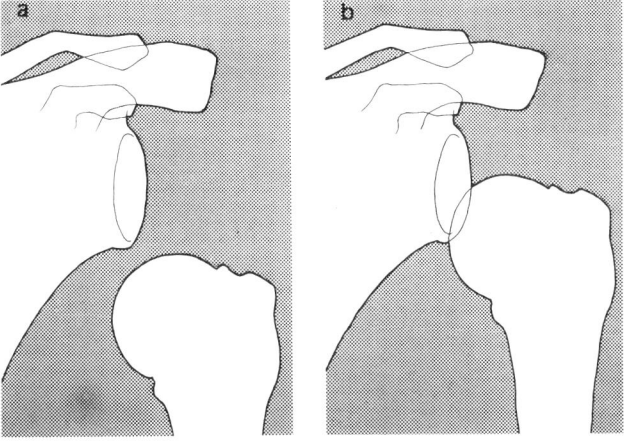

FIG. 3.3. (a) Dislocation. (b) Subluxation.

If there is still some contact between the articular surfaces the displacement is referred to as a subluxation (Fig. 3.3).

It may help you to remember these terms if we point out that in the 1800s, the term 'luxation' was used for complete displacement and 'subluxation' for incomplete displacement. For some unknown reason we have dropped one (luxation) but kept the other (subluxation).

Signs
1. Deformity.
2. Tenderness.
3. Reduction of range of movement where previously there had been movement. (Compare with signs of a fracture, p. 15. In a fracture there is increased mobility.)

Treatment
The principles are similar to those for treatment of a fracture.
1. The dislocation is reduced.
2. The joint is then immobilized until the capsule and ligaments have undergone repair.
3. The joint is then protected until a full range of movement is regained.

Complications
1. Damage to other structures at the time of injury, e.g. nerves.
2. Stiffness of the joint following injury, especially in older people.
3. Laxity of the capsule and recurrent dislocation if mobilization is started too early, especially in young people.

4 The management of the severely injured patient

It is inevitable that during his period of duty in the Accident and Emergency Department, the Casualty Officer will be called upon to deal with severely injured patients. It is essential that he automatically applies a system of priorities to the investigation he makes or he will run the risk of the patient suffering irreversible damage from injury to one system, while the Casualty Officer is busy investigating another, less immediately important, system.

Death occurring within the first few hours following an accident is caused by tissue anoxia and this is due to either inadequate oxygenation of the blood in the lungs or inadequate circulation of the blood to the tissues. The assessment of the severely injured patient should therefore proceed in the following sequence:
1. *Airway*. Check that the airway is clear.
2. *Breathing*. Check that the chest is moving normally and that air entry to each lung is satisfactory.
3. *Circulation*. Check the pulse rate, blood-pressure, and state of the skin circulation in the extremities.
4. *Injuries*. Check the head, neck, shoulder girdle, chest, abdomen, pelvis, and limbs for signs of injuries.

Note that these priorities are in alphabetical order, A, B, C, I, which helps one to remember them in an emergency.

AIRWAY

The commonest causes of airway obstruction are:
(1) falling back of the jaw with resultant closing of the oro-pharynx by the back of the tongue pressing against the back of the pharynx;
(2) dentures becoming dislodged;
(3) foreign bodies present in the air passages;
(4) blood and mucus in the air passages.

These causes can usually be rapidly diagnosed and dealt with. Occasionally laryngoscopy is necessary to inspect the larynx. The ability to pass an endotracheal tube is essential to those dealing with trauma.

BREATHING

Paradoxical breathing

The excursion of the chest wall during breathing should be observed. One part of the rib cage may not move in unison with the rest; when the chest cage as a whole expands, this area is drawn in and when the chest cage contracts this area is pushed out. This is referred to as 'paradoxical movement' and implies that there is a flail segment of the chest wall. As a first-aid measure this segment should be held still by means of a pad held in place manually. The best method of long-term management is the use of a positive-pressure aeration system to fill the lungs and hence to avoid the 'sucking in' of the flail segment which is due to the negative intrathoracic pressure present during active inspiration.

Tension pneumothorax

This condition arises if there is damage to the lung which causes it to act as a one-way valve allowing air to be sucked from the air passages into the pleural space during inspiration, but preventing its return to the air passages during expiration. The amount of air in the pleural space builds up and compresses the damaged lung. Its pressure may become high enough to force the mediastinum to move towards the other side of the chest. Diminished air entry, increased resonance to percussion, and displacement of the apex beat towards the unaffected side of the chest are findings indicative of a tension pneumothorax.

Treatment

The pressure of air in the affected pleural cavity should be reduced as soon as possible because of the danger of cardiac and respiratory embarrassment. A wide-bore cannula should be introduced between two of the upper ribs in the mid-clavicular line and connected to an underwater-seal drain. As the trochar is withdrawn from the cannula, the air is expelled with an audible hiss. It is important to prevent re-entry of air once the pressure in the pleural cavity has been reduced. If the underwater-seal drain is not immediately available the tubing attached to the cannula should be temporarily clamped.

It is customary to maintain underwater-seal drainage to the pleural cavity for several days to allow the lung injury to heal and the lung to re-expand.

Having established that the airway is clear and that the patient is breathing satisfactorily, attention is turned to the cardiovascular system.

THE CARDIOVASCULAR SYSTEM

Adequate perfusion of the vital organs of the body depends on three factors:
1. The volume of circulating blood. It must not be depleted.
2. The tone of the vascular tree, which must be such that the blood at the arterial end of the capillary bed is under adequate hydrostatic pressure.
3. Satisfactory pumping of the heart.

In cases of severe trauma it is usually the first and second factors which are threatened and if the circulation through the tissues and organs becomes inadequate the patient is said to be in a state of cardiovascular decompensation or 'shock'.

Shock

Commonly the clinical sign of impending shock is that the pulse rate rises. If no treatment is given, this is followed by a fall in the blood-pressure. The skin becomes cold and clammy and the patient becomes very apprehensive. If the blood-pressure is allowed to remain low, two complications may arise:
1. The myocardium may become ischaemic, and this may lead to arrhythmias or cardiac arrest.

2. Renal ischaemia may lead to damage to the parenchymal cells and subsequent renal failure.

Causes
1. *Loss of circulating blood volume.* An adult can lose half a litre of blood without obvious effect on pulse or blood-pressure. Any larger amount will lead to signs of shock. This loss of blood may be obvious if bleeding to the exterior occurs. Of particular danger is bleeding into the body cavities—especially the thorax and abdomen—and into the tissues. It is usual for a closed fracture of the femur to be associated with a loss of a litre of blood into the thigh or a severe fracture of the pelvis to be associated with a loss of 2 litres of blood into the retroperitoneal tissues. This bleeding may continue for a long period and lead to circulatory collapse several hours after the patient's admission to hospital.

2. *Loss of vascular tone.* If the normal degree of vasoconstriction of the vascular tree is lost, the pressure of the enclosed blood will fall and tissue perfusion will then become inadequate. This phenomenon is seen if severe neurological stimuli are suffered by the patient. The commonest stimulus encountered in trauma is severe pain—as seen, for example, when fractured bones are allowed to move unsplinted. The resultant drop in blood-pressure may be associated with slowing of the pulse rate—the so-called vasovagal syndrome.

The adrenocortical hormones are necessary for the normal preservation of vascular tone, and a prolonged strain on the cardiovascular system may lead to a drop in blood-pressure because of a deficiency in these hormones.

Severe toxaemia or septicaemia may also cause loss of vascular tone.

3. *Heart failure.* This is rarely the primary cause of the shock seen in traumatic states. However, if the blood-pressure remains low for some other reason, the myocardium may be inadequately oxygenated and, itself, become a factor in the shock state. This is particularly likely if the heart was previously diseased.

The myocardium may also be affected by toxaemia or septicaemia.

Prevention and treatment
The object of treatment is to keep the blood-pressure at a level sufficient to guarantee adequate tissue perfusion. In practical terms this means, in normal individuals, a systolic pressure of over 90 mm Hg and, in the previously hypertensive patient, a systolic pressure above his pre-accident diatolic pressure.

1. *Restoration of circulating volume.* Any loss of blood must be replaced as soon as possible. The best fluid for replacement is blood itself but, as cross-matching the blood may take some time, a substitute—plasma or dextran—may be used. The substitute fluid must have a large molecular weight so that it remains where it is needed, in the vascular tree, and does not diffuse out into the interstitial fluid compartment. Samples of the patient's blood for cross-matching should be taken before dextran is administered, because its effect is to cause increased rouleaux formation and it may therefore interfere with cross-matching.

Since the heart cannot pump out more blood than is presented to it (the venous return) this amount should be kept adequate but not allowed to exceed the capabilities of the heart. A fall in the venous return is accompanied by a drop in the hydrostatic pressure in the great veins on the right side of the heart (the superior and inferior venae cavae) and an excessive venous return causes a rise in this pressure.

To monitor this central venous pressure, a long intravenous catheter is passed into the cubital vein and via the axillary and subclavian veins into the superior vena cava. By attaching this tube to a manometer the central venous pressure can be measured. The usual aim is to keep the central venous pressure between 3 cm H_2O and 10 cm H_2O.

It is also advisable to monitor the ECG tracing of the patient so that early signs of arrhythmias can be noted.

A temporary increase in the venous return can be produced by tipping the patient into 10–20° of the Trendelenberg (head-down) position, hence increasing the return of blood from the lower extremities.

2. *The maintenance of vascular tone.* Adequate analgesia must be produced and all fractures reduced and immobilized as quickly as possible.

The diagnosis of adrenocortical insufficiency should only be made when the other causes of shock have been excluded. It is treated by the administration of intravenous hydrocortisone.

Toxaemia and septicaemia require specific treatment with appropriate antibiotics and antitoxins.

INJURIES

A thorough search for injuries should be made. Those commonly overlooked are:

1. *Skull fractures.* The skull should be X-rayed in all cases in which there has been any injury to the head or any history of unconsciousness.
2. *Cervical spine dislocations.* These tend to be overlooked in cases also suffering from head injuries, especially if unconscious.
3. *Intra-abdominal bleeding.* Again more difficult to diagnose in the unconscious patient.
4. *Fractures around the ankles and toes.*

It is a good working plan to re-examine the patient on the morning following his admission to hospital in the same manner as one would on initial examination. In my experience this practice brings to light a significant number of further injuries which were not diagnosed on first assessment. This is seen particularly in patients who are unconscious on admission to hospital.

RECOMMENDATIONS FOR FURTHER READING

BICKFORD, B. J. (1973) Chest injuries. In *Basic Clinical Surgery for Nurses and Medical Students* (ed. J. McFarland), Chapter 15, Butterworths, London.

GERSON, G. R. (1973) Shock. In *Intensive Care*, Heinemann, London.

GILBERTSON, A. A. (1973) Respiratory failure. In *Basic Clinical Surgery for Nurses and Medical Students* (ed. J. McFarland), Chapter 5, Butterworths, London.

JONES, P. F. (1974) Abdominal injuries. In *Emergency Abdominal Surgery*, Chapter 17, Blackwell, Oxford.

SEDZIMIR, C. B. (1973) Head injuries. In *Basic Clinical Surgery for Nurses and Medical Students* (ed. J. McFarland), Chapter 13, Butterworths, London.

5 Conditions affecting peripheral nerves

The spinal peripheral nerves are formed by the junction of the motor and sensory roots near the spinal cord. Cranial nerves may be considered as peripheral nerves from the point of leaving the brain stem.

Three main groups of conditions affecting peripheral nerves will be described:
  (1) traumatic conditions (peripheral nerve injuries);
  (2) the 'tunnel' syndromes of nerve construction;
  (3) the varieties of neurofibromatoses.

PERIPHERAL NERVE INJURIES

Three grades of nerve injury occur:
1. *Neurapraxia.* The nerve is contused but there is no interruption of anatomical continuity of the axons.
2. *Neurotmesis.* There is complete division of the nerve.
3. *Axonotmesis.* Although the nerve is intact, the axons have been 'snapped'. The myelin sheath is intact so recovery is possible.

Cause

Compression of a nerve is the common cause of neurapraxia. This may be due to the edge of splints or plaster casts pressing on the nerve, or to the limb lying over a sharp edge, e.g. radial palsy following sleeping with the arm over the back of a chair (Saturday night palsy).

Neurotmesis is usually caused by sharp objects, e.g. a knife or splinter of glass from without or a sharp spicule of bone from within.

Axonotmesis is also seen in nerve injuries complicating fractures.

Symptoms

The patient notices an inability to use the muscles innervated by the injured nerve or an area of numbness corresponding to the area of supply of the nerve.

Signs

The findings are those of a lower motor neurone lesion:
  (1) weakness or paralysis of muscles supplied;
  (2) loss or diminution of tendon jerks of muscles supplied;
  (3) loss of tone of muscles supplied;
  (4) loss or diminution of sensation over the area of skin supplied by the nerve.

Special investigations
Electromyography may show loss of resting activity in the muscle. Nerve conduction studies show partial or complete interruption of conduction. The strength/duration curve shows contraction of the muscle in the high voltage/long duration part of the graph.

Common clinical types
Although any peripheral nerve may be damaged, the following clinical types are commonly seen.

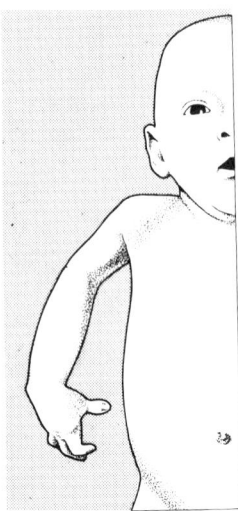

FIG. 5.1. The position adopted by a baby with an Erb's palsy: the 'Waiter's tip' position.

Facial paralysis
This follows swelling of the tissues in the facial canal. Paralysis of the muscles of expression on the same side follows. The eye cannot be closed and the corner of the mouth droops. Treatment is by splintage to prevent unnatural distortion of the face. Most cases recover but recovery may not be complete.

Brachial plexus injuries
The plexus may be damaged by direct trauma, e.g. in cases of assault, but more commonly damage follows traction lesions caused by falls from fast-moving vehicles, e.g. motor cycles, in which the shoulder and neck are rapidly forced apart. The diagnosis may not be immediately apparent because of a concomitant head injury. The plexus may also be damaged during delivery of a difficult breech presentation.
Four main patterns of neurological deficit are commonly seen.
1. *The upper plexus lesion (Erb's palsy).* In this type the nerves arising from the fifth and sixth cervical roots are affected. The muscles denervated are the shoulder abductors, the elbow flexors, the wrist extensors, and the supinators. The limb takes up the characteristic 'waiter's tip' position: adducted at the shoulder, extended at the elbow, pronated and flexed at the wrist (Fig. 5.1).
2. *The medial cord lesion.* In this type the branches of the medial cord (that cord which lies medial to the axillary artery) suffers damage with resultant loss of action of the ulnar nerve, the medial cutaneous nerve of arm and forearm, the medial pectoral nerve, and the medial root of the median nerve. The clinical presentation is that of an ulnar palsy with some loss of median function—usually finger flexion—and sensory loss on the medial side of the arm, forearm, and hand.
3. *The lower plexus lesion (Klumpke's palsy).* In this the nerves taking origin from the eighth cervical and first thoracic segments are damaged. Neurological deficit is mainly in the small muscles of the hand.
4. *The total plexus lesion.* In this type all the nerves arising from the fifth cervical to the first thoracic root are damaged. The whole of the upper limb is paralysed.
Erb's and Klumpke's palsies are often seen as birth injuries.

Conditions affecting peripheral nerves 27

Prognosis. Damage to the roots as they leave the spinal cord leads to permanent loss of function. Distal to this the plexus consists of peripheral nerve fibres and so some recovery is possible.

The level of the lesion may be estimated by the histamine response. This is an axon reflex which requires an intact sensory neurone. If there is continuity between the cell body in the dorsal root ganglion and the skin receptor endings, an intracuticular injection of a minute amount of histamine will cause a wheal. This implies that the lesion is between the sensory (dorsal) root ganglion and the spinal cord, i.e. no recovery is possible. However, if the histamine response in the paralysed limb is negative, the lesion is in the 'peripheral nerve' part of the plexus and some recovery may occur.

Introduction of radio-opaque dye into the cervical subarachnoid space (myelography) may show empty root sleeves in the dura of the affected segments, again signifying a poor prognosis for recovery.

Treatment. Most authorities agree that exploration and repair of the damaged nerves does little to improve the prognosis.

The completely flail arm with no prospect of recovery is best treated by amputation through the humerus after fusion of the shoulder to facilitate manipulation of an arm prosthesis.

Radial nerve paralysis
This is caused by direct injury, e.g. complicating a fracture of the humerus, or by pressure as mentioned on p. 25. The effects are loss of power of extension of the m.p. joints of the fingers and the dorsiflexors of the wrist. Sensory loss is minimal—occasionally a small area of anaesthesia over the dorsum of the index finger metacarpal is found.

Ulnar nerve paralysis
Damage to the ulnar nerve usually occurs at the elbow. It may be due to stretching, as seen in fractures of the capitellum or, less acutely, with the development of a valgus deformity at the elbow.

The motor effects are weakness of the ulnar flexor of the wrist and weakness of the intrinsic muscles of the hand, with the exception of the thenar muscles and the lumbrical muscles to the index and middle fingers. This leads to a characteristic deformity: the metacarpo-phalangeal joints of the ring and little

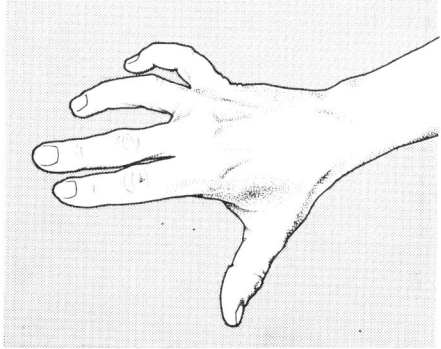

FIG. 5.2. The 'ulnar claw' hand.

fingers are hyperextended and the interphalangeal joints of these fingers are flexed (ulnar or half claw hand; Fig. 5.2). There is also loss of power of abduction and adduction of the fingers. Wasting of the interossei may be present. It is usually most obvious between the thumb and index finger. The sensory loss affects the ulnar border of the palm (front and back), the little finger, and the ulnar half of the ring finger.

Froment's sign. This sign demonstrates weakness of the adductor pollicis muscle—usually due to ulnar nerve paralysis or paresis. When asked to hold a thin piece of cardboard in the space between the thumb and the radial border of the palm a person with a normal hand does so by adducting the thumb and keeping the interphalangeal joint of the thumb extended. The person with a weak adductor pollicis holds the card by flexing the interphalangeal joint of the thumb using flexor pollicis longus. This constitutes a positive Froment's sign.

The ulnar nerve may also be damaged in the arm or forearm. The level of the lesion determines the degree of loss of function and subsequent deformity. The higher the level of the lesion the greater the loss of function but, surprisingly enough, the less the degree of deformity. This is because a functioning flexor digitorum profundus is necessary for the formation of the 'claw' deformity—if the ulnar nerve is divided proximal to the point at which it supplies flexor digitorum profundus, the claw deformity does not develop. This is referred to as the 'ulnar paradox'.

Median nerve paralysis
The median nerve is usually damaged at the wrist or at the elbow. Total damage at either site causes anaesthesia of the palmar surfaces of the index, middle, and ring fingers, the thumb, and the radial half of the palm. The thenar muscles are paralysed but adduction of the thumb is retained. If the damage is at the wrist level the long flexors of the fingers are not paralysed. Damage at the elbow denervates the flexor digitorum profundus to the index finger and, to a certain extent, those fibres acting on the middle finger. This causes the characteristic position of the fingers at rest—flexion of the little and ring fingers, partial flexion of the middle finger, and a straight index finger ('the pointing index of median nerve paralysis').

Division of ulnar and median nerves at the wrist causes 'clawing' of all four fingers ('total claw hand').

Sciatic nerve injuries
These are seen following dislocations of the hip and penetrating wounds of the thigh.

If the nerve is damaged in the buttock, motor loss affects the knee flexors and all muscles below the knee, while sensory loss affects the whole of the foot and leg up to the knee with the exception of the medial side of shin and calf.

Lateral popliteal nerve
This is the nerve most prone to injury in the lower limb. The motor effects are loss of dorsiflexion and eversion of the ankle and toes (i.e. drop-foot). Plantar flexion of the foot is not affected. There is sensory loss over the peroneal region of the leg and the dorsum of the foot and toes.

Treatment

Except in the case of very small nerves which are technically not reparable, all divided nerves should be sutured. Most authorities recommend a delay of 3–6 weeks after the injury before attempting nerve suture. This gives time for the original skin laceration to heal and for any infection to be controlled. It is also easier to suture a nerve at this time because the sheath has become thicker and more fibrous. The fibrous 'neuromata' at the cut end of the nerve can be excised and co-aption of healthy Schwann sheaths can be obtained.

In a clean-cut injury, however, some authorities advocate nerve suture at the time of the injury.

It is sometimes difficult in closed injuries to decide whether neurotmesis or a lesser degree of injury has occurred. In these cases it is reasonable to wait for a period of up to 6–8 weeks to see whether any recovery takes place before exploring the nerve.

While recovery is awaited the joints distal to the injury should be kept mobile by periodically moving them through a full range of movement. Electrical stimulation of paralysed muscles keeps them supple and maintains the patient's morale.

'TUNNEL' OR CONSTRICTION SYNDROMES OF PERIPHERAL NERVES

Ulnar neuritis

Compression at the elbow

The ulnar nerve may be compressed at the elbow by a fibrous tunnel as it passes deep to flexor carpi ulnaris.

Symptoms. The patient complains of numbness or paraesthesia over the ulnar border of the hand and the ring and little fingers. Clumsiness is also noticed.

Signs. The ulnar claw hand may be present as may wasting of the interossei. This is best seen in the first dorsal interosseus, a dent appearing between the index and thumb metacarpals. The spaces between the other metacarpals on the dorsum of the hand may also be 'furrowed'.

Froment's sign may be positive and weakness of finger abduction and adduction is weak compared with the normal side.

Treatment. The nerve may be decompressed at the elbow or transposed to the flexor compartment of the forearm so that it comes to lie anterior to the medial humeral epicondyle and is less likely to be stretched.

Compression at the wrist

Another type of ulnar neuritis deserves mention. Occasionally the nerve is compressed by a ganglion at the wrist. The hand symptoms and signs are the same as those due to compression at the elbow with the exception of the area of paraesthesia and hypoaesthesia to testing. In cases of compression at the wrist, the dorsal aspect of the ulnar side of the hand is spared as the branch of the ulnar nerve supplying this comes off the main nerve well above the wrist. There is therefore no area of numbness on the dorsum of the hand and fingers.

30 Orthopaedics for Undergraduates

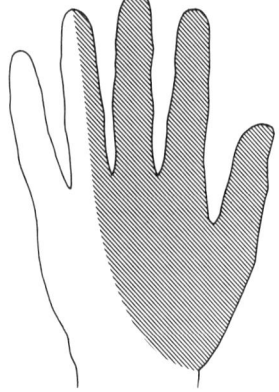

FIG. 5.3. The area of tingling in the carpal tunnel syndrome.

Carpal tunnel syndrome

Cause
The carpal tunnel syndrome results from compression of the median nerve as it passes under the flexor retinaculum at the wrist. This retinaculum is a strong fibrous structure attaching to the trapezium and scaphoid laterally, and the hook of the hamate and pisiform medially. The syndrome is seen most commonly in middle-aged women, but also in any condition reducing the volume of the tunnel, e.g. fractures of the lunate. It may also cause troublesome symptoms in pregnancy.

Symptoms
Tingling in the thumb, index finger, and middle fingers is characteristic (Fig. 5.3). This tingling often wakens the patient at night (about 2 a.m.) and she obtains relief by shaking the hand. There may be weakness of the thumb and clumsiness on attempted delicate movements.

Signs
The thenar eminence may be wasted. Sensation over the palmar aspects of the thumb and index and mid-fingers may be diminished. The tingling in the fingers may be brought on by rendering the limb ischaemic. This is achieved by applying a sphygmomanometer cuff to the arm and inflating it to 200 mm Hg. The symptoms come on after about 0·5–1·5 minutes and, to constitute a positive 'tourniquet test' should affect only the digits innervated by the median nerve. Occasionally the tingling is brought on by inflating the cuff to about 60 mm Hg, thus producing engorgement of the limb. Again, for the test to be positive, the symptoms must be confined to the thumb, index finger, and middle finger.

The diagnosis may be confirmed in doubtful cases by asking the patient to wear a wrist splint at night; if this immobilization cures the symptoms and prevents the patient from waking, this is confirmatory evidence of the presence of the carpal tunnel syndrome.

Treatment
Mild cases may respond to local injection of hydrocortisone acetate into the carpal tunnel. In the type occurring in pregnancy the majority of cases respond to diuretics, suggesting that water retention may be the cause.

Complete relief of symptoms usually follows operative division of the ligament.

Meralgia paraesthetica

Cause
This results from compression of the lateral cutaneous nerve of the thigh in a fascial envelope at the level of its emergence either through or under the inguinal ligament.

Symptoms
Paraesthesia is felt over the antero-lateral part of the right thigh.

Signs
An area of hypoaesthesia or anaesthesia, which corresponds to the area of supply of the nerve, is found on testing sensation to pin-prick. The area extends from just below the inguinal ligament, down the antero-lateral part of the thigh to just above the knee.

Treatment
Operative decompression of the nerve is usually required to relieve the symptoms.

Tarsal tunnel syndrome

This syndrome has only recently been described and is comparatively rare.

Cause
Compression of the posterior tibial nerve behind and below the medial malleolus.

Symptoms
A warm feeling under the medial side of the sole of the foot.

Signs
Hypoaesthesia in an area usually corresponding to the area of distribution of the medial plantar nerve.

Treatment
Operative decompression is recommended.

NEUROFIBROMATOSIS

This is the only common neoplastic condition affecting peripheral nerves. Although the degree of interrelationship is still in doubt it is probably justifiable to consider the following as subdivisions of the same group.

1. *Multiple neurofibromatosis* (von Recklinghausen's disease of nerves). Multiple small firm swellings are found in the subcutaneous tissues in any or all parts of the body. Areas of skin pigmentation may be found in these cases.
2. *Plexiform neurofibromatosis.* This condition is characterized by massive soft subcutaneous tumours, often localized to one limb, which causes stretching of the overlying skin so that it hangs down in folds.
3. *Acoustic neuroma.* A localized swelling occurring on the eighth cranial nerve in its intracranial course. Deafness, tinnitus, and cerebellar signs may be caused.

4. *Elephantiasis neuromatosa.* In this condition the subcutaneous tissue and skin, usually of one limb, shows tremendous overgrowth.
5. *Dumb-bell tumour of the spine.* A small tumour within the spinal canal connected by an isthmus in the intervertebral foramen with a large tumour in the paraspinal area. Pain and long-tract signs are common.

Histology

This reveals varying proportions of tissue derived from the Schwann cell sheath and from the fibrous covering of the nerve.

Associated anomalies

Neurofibromata are often found in association with other orthopaedic conditions, particularly scoliosis, spina bifida, and pseudarthrosis of the tibia. The neurofibromata may be present within the bone substance and cause cystic spaces visible at operation and on radiographs.

Treatment

When symptoms or signs attributable to the presence of a neurofibroma arise, e.g. in the dumb-bell tumours of the spine, the tumour should be removed. Massive tumours of the limbs may justify amputation.

Prognosis

Sarcomatous degeneration does occur on rare occasions.

6 Rheumatoid disease

Rheumatoid disease usually presents as a subacute inflammation of joints and tendon sheaths which characteristically shows remissions and relapses, and often revolves spontaneously. Some cases, however, show a gradual progressive course leading to complete disorganization of the affected joint and the development of deformities. The disease tends to affect more than one joint and usually starts in the small joints of the hands and feet.

Pathology

Joints
The disease process starts in the synovial membrane, which becomes swollen and hyperaemic. Cellular infiltration, mainly by lymphocytes and plasma cells, is seen.

An edge of this inflammatory tissue (referred to as a 'pannus') spreads over the articular surfaces of the joint and the articular cartilage under it undergoes degenerative ulceration. This, of course, predisposes to the development of degenerative arthrosis in later life.

The hypertrophic synovium distends and stretches the capsule and ligaments of the joint. When a remission occurs and the synovium returns to normal size, the lax ligaments allow deformities of the joint to occur.

Tendon sheaths
The synovial membrane becomes hypertrophic and hyperaemic and tends to adhere to the tendon. This swelling of the synovium may cause a clinically palpable and visible swelling along the line of the tendon. The enclosed tendon may undergo attrition and finally rupture. Characteristically, this occurs in the long extensors of the fingers.

Skin
Rheumatoid nodules occur commonly—they are most often seen on the dorsal aspect of the elbow and forearm. Histologically these consist of a central area of necrotic collagen fibres surrounded by palisades of fibroblasts with areas of round cell infiltration.

Stills disease; Felty's syndrome
Regional lymphadenitis may occur and occasionally hepatomegaly and splenomegaly are also seen. If seen in childhood this combination is referred to as Still's disease; if accompanied by leucopaenia it constitutes Felty's syndrome.

Symptoms

The earliest symptom is stiffness of the joints. This is usually first seen in the finger joints and most noticed by the patient in the early mornings. Later pain

34 *Orthopaedics for Undergraduates*

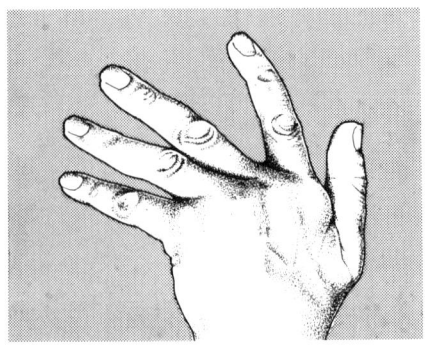

FIG. 6.1.
Ulnar deviation of the fingers.

and swelling of the affected joints or tendon sheaths is noted. The disease shows characteristic exacerbations and remissions, the patient suffering from malaise and often fever during the exacerbations.

Signs
The patient may be pale. The affected joints are swollen—the combination of synovial swelling and extra-capsular thickening result in a characteristic spindle shape of the joints involved.

In the hand an early sign of metacarpo-phalangeal joint involvement is the 'filling-in' of the normal grooves between the metacarpal heads as seen from their dorsal aspect.

Later in the disease the fingers may take on a characteristic ulnar deviation at the metacarpo-phalangeal joints (Fig. 6.1) often associated with either flexion or extension deformities of the interphalangeal joints. These give rise to the 'swan-neck' (Fig. 6.2) and 'boutonnière' (Fig. 6.3) deformities.

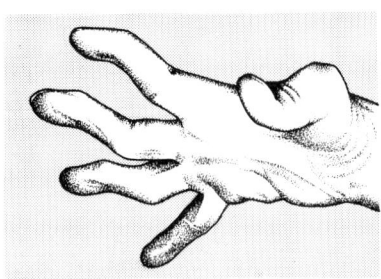

FIG. 6.2.
The 'swan neck' deformity of the fingers.

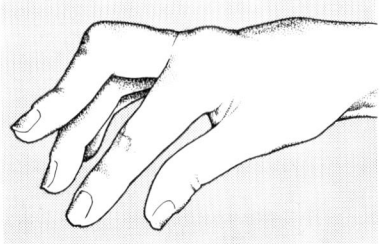

FIG. 6.3.
The 'boutonnière' deformity of the finger.

Rheumatoid disease 35

The knees are commonly affected—synovial effusions and later degenerative changes are seen. Characteristically a valgus deformity occurs.

Radiographs
These show general decrease in bone density with subperiosteal erosions in the phalanges—the ulnar styloid is characteristically eroded. At a later stage in the disease, the changes of degenerative arthritis are seen in addition to those of rheumatoid arthritis.

Special tests
1. *Erythrocyte sedimentation rate*
This is usually raised during the acute phase.
2. *Detection of the rheumatoid factor*
The rheumatoid factor is a macroglobulin, an antibody to 7s globulin, and causes agglutination of red cells coated with globulin (the Rose–Waaler test) or of latex coated with 7s human globulin (the latex agglutination test).
   These tests are often negative during the early stages of the disease.

Treatment
Relief of pain
Different patients obtain relief using different analgesics. The most commonly effective are salicylates, phenylbutazone, and indomethacin. They all have irritative effects on the gastric mucosa and this may preclude their use, especially in patients suffering from peptic ulceration. With phenylbutazone therapy it is important to monitor the white cell count because of the danger of agranulocytosis.

Suppression of inflammatory responses
Steroids may have marked effects in relieving pain and stiffness but most clinicians feel that their long-term side effects—electrolyte inbalance, osteoporosis, moon-face, hypertension, and reduced glucose tolerance—outweigh their usefulness in rheumatoid disease.

Local treatment
Splintage of painful joints during the acute stage and mobilization of pain-free joints is the accepted treatment.
   Intra-articular injection of steroids under strict aseptic conditions is beneficial in individual joints but should not be given more than three times into any one joint because of the danger of joint degeneration.
   Synovectomy has good results if carried out before articular cartilage ulceration has occurred.
   Arthroplasty is highly successful in selected cases. Finger joints, hip joints, and knee joints can be satisfactorily replaced using plastic or metal replacement prostheses.
   Arthrodesis of painful or disorganized joints carries a high success rate. It is particularly applicable to the metacarpo-phalangeal joints and the knee joint.

7 Cerebral palsy and poliomyelitis

CEREBRAL PALSY

This term is used to denote a large number of conditions developing in infancy and early childhood, all attributable to lesions in the central nervous system.

Causes
There are many causes, the commonest of which can be classified as to the time of occurrence:
1. *Before birth.* Foetal distress, toxaemia of pregnancy, rhesus incompatability antepartum haemorrhage.
2. *During birth.* Foetal anoxia and birth trauma.
3. *After birth.* Neonatal jaundice, meningitis, encephalitis, and head injuries.

Pathology
Opportunities for pathological examination of the central nervous system are rare but those which do occur they suggest that there is still evidence to support the standard teaching: in the spastic type the lesions are predominently in the motor cortex; in the athetoid type the lesions are in the basal ganglia, and in the ataxic type it is the cerebellum that is mainly affected (Table 7.1).

TABLE 7.1. *Types of cerebral palsy*

Type	Proportion of total cases (percentage)
Spastic type	70
Athetoid type	10
Ataxic type	10
Atonic and mixed type	10

Clinical features
In childhood

It is important to diagnose cerebral palsy as early as possible, and in the first few months of life the diagnosis should be considered when there is any delay of development from reflex to voluntary activity or any other motor abnormality.
Common abnormalities are:
  difficulty with sucking or swallowing;
  development of a squint;
  delay in control of eyes in response to a stimulus;

Cerebral palsy and poliomyelitis

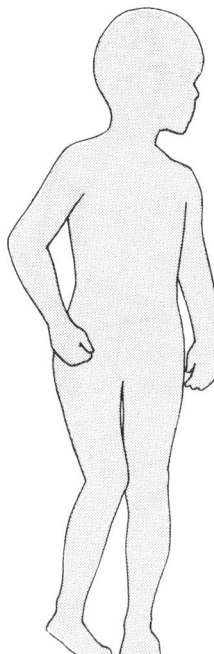

FIG. 7.1. Typical stance of a child with spastic hemiplegia.

delay in holding head up (usually about 3 months);
delay in sitting up (usually about 6 months);
delay in standing (usually 9–12 months);
delay in walking (usually 12–15 months);
delay in speaking recognizable words (usually 14–20 months).
Spasm of muscles or increased tone may be noted, e.g. hip adductor spasm causing difficulty with putting on nappies.

Later signs
As the child grows, more obvious muscular abnormalities may be noted:
    loss of co-ordination in upper or lower limbs;
    athetoid movements;
    spastic hip adductors leading to 'scissor-gait';
    flexion contractures of knees;
    equinus contractures of ankles;
    flexion contracture of elbows and wrists;
    pronation contractures of forearms;
    adduction contracture of the thumb,

The muscular abnormalities may be present in:
    one limb (monoplegia);
    upper and lower limb on the same side (hemiplegia);
    both lower limbs (paraplegia);
    all four limbs (quadriplegia);
    all four limbs but lower limbs more severely affected than upper limbs (diplegia).

Associated abnormalities
About 75 per cent of these children are mentally retarded, 33 per cent are subject to fits, and 20 per cent have some degree of deafness. Visual defects and speech and emotional disorders are also common.

General treatment
Special educational facilities, speech therapy, and psychological handling may be necessary. The child should be encouraged to use any skills he may possess, no matter how bizarre his pattern of movement.

Orthopaedic treatment
This has two main objects:
    (1) keeping the patient as ambulant as possible;
    (2) preventing contractures, deformities, and dislocations.
Walking exercises, encouragement, and psychotherapy are the most important ways of keeping the patient ambulant.
    Deformities, contractures, and dislocations are usually due to unequal muscle pull, e.g. the equinus at the ankle being caused by an overactive calf muscle and weak dorsiflexors of the ankle.

In mild cases and in the early stages in severe cases, deformities and contractures can be prevented by periodical stretching of the affected muscles and the application of supporting splints to be worn either continuously or in some cases, at night only.

Methods of correcting muscle imbalance
1. *Interference with nerve supply of overacting muscles.* This is now virtually confined to partial obturator neurectomy for overacting hip adductors.
2. *Tenotomy or lengthening of tendons of overacting muscles.* (a) Adductor tenotomy at the hip; (b) hamstring tenotomy for overacting knee flexors; (c) lengthening of the tendo-Achilles for equinus deformities.
3. *Transplanting tendons to alter their actions.* Examples include (a) hamstring tendons detached from back of tibia and attached to back of femur, hence converting them from knee flexors to hip extensors (Egger's operation); (b) tibialis posterior transplant from sole of the foot to the dorsum, hence converting from plantar flexor to dorsiflexor.

It is important after these operations to keep the patients under review until growth is complete because transferring tendons may, as the child grows, produce an opposite deformity.

The child should be examined periodically throughout the growing period and special attention paid to the above-mentioned common sites of deformity. In addition, the spine should be examined for scoliosis, the hips for subluxation, and the heels for valgus or varus deformities.

When growth is complete arthrodesis of joints, especially the wrist and sub-talar joints, may be undertaken in order to increase the patient's control of the hand or foot.

It is important that the patient as a whole—his mental as well as physical potential—should always be considered with the ultimate aim of making him as useful a member of society as his disabilities will allow.

POLIOMYELITIS

There has been a virtual disappearance of poliomyelitis as an acute infectious disease since the introduction of the vaccine, but in orthopaedics we still encounter the late results and, very occasionally, a new case from abroad.

The poliomyelitis virus selectively attacks the anterior horn cell of the spinal cord causing a motor paralysis of the lower motor neurone type. The sensory paths of the central nervous system are not involved and these patients therefore have no impairment of sensation.

Clinical features

The signs of a lower motor neurone lesion are all present—weakness, wasting, loss of tone, diminished tendon reflexes, and the plantar flexor response.

The commonest muscles affected in the lower limb are the dorsiflexors of toes and ankle (leading to the drop-foot gait) but weak knee extensors, calf muscles, and glutei (causing a positive Trendelenburg sign and/or weak hip extension) are also seen. Upper limb muscles may also be weak or paralysed, the shoulder abductors and finger flexors being commonly affected. The weakness of lower limb muscles, if extensive, may cause retardation in growth, the child ending the growth period with the affected limb shorter than the normal one.

The orthopaedic surgeon has to concern himself with three aspects of poliomyelitis:
(1) muscle imbalance, leading to reduced function or deformity of the limbs;
(2) limb-length discrepancy;
(3) scoliosis—this will be of the neuropathic or paralytic type.

Muscle imbalance
Disability due to weakness is best treated by building up by physiotherapy any muscle fibres that remain functional, and later reinforcing this action by means of tendon transplantation to allow normal muscles (if they can be spared from their normal function) to act in a different way.

Examples of tendon transplants used in this way are:
(1) transplantation of the hamstrings into the quadriceps expansion to help knee extension;
(2) transplantation of tibialis posterior through the interosseus membrane of the leg to the dorsum of the foot to help ankle dorsiflexion;
(3) transplantation of wrist flexors to the dorsal aspect of the wrist to help wrist extension.

Limb-length discrepancy
Poliomyelitis is the commonest cause of shortening encountered in modern practice, the other causes being damage to the epiphyseal plate, fractures, chronic hip disease, and congenital shortening.

There are two ways of dealing with leg-length discrepancy—either to shorten the longer limb or lengthen the shorter one. Since shortening the longer limb usually means operating on a normal limb most surgeons (and patients) prefer the lengthening of the shorter limb. It must be pointed out, however, that the shortening of a femur is a relatively simple and very successful procedure.

Femoral lengthening. This procedure is becoming more popular now that the technical difficulties are being overcome. Up to 5 cm of lengthening can be obtained. Two techniques are in use: the first involves the gradual distraction of an osteotomy using transverse pinning and a special extending frame, and the second uses an intermedullary nail to hold alignment after transverse osteotomy while the two femoral segments are distracted by skeletal traction.

Tibial lengthening. This is the procedure more commonly carried out. Two transverse Steinmann pins are inserted into each section of the tibia, which is then osteotomized at a point about its centre. The fibula must be osteotomized at the same time. The pins are then attached to a distraction frame and the osteotomy distracted at the rate of 1 mm per day. When the required lengthening has been obtained distraction is held at that point until new bone has been laid down by the stretched periosteum. The distraction frame is then dismantled and the limb immobilized in a plaster of Paris cast until the osteotomy site has consolidated.

There are two disadvantages of tibial lengthening:
1. Distortion of the ankle may occur because the fibula is not as amenable to lengthening as the tibia. This distortion is avoided by a preliminary opera- which separates the lower third of the fibula from the rest of the bone.

2. A fixed equinus deformity may develop at the ankle due to the fact that the calf does not elongate as effectively as the anterior group of tibial muscles. The deformity can be minimized by elongating the tendo-Achilles and other flexor tendons at the ankle prior to the tibial lengthening procedure. The maximum amount of lengthening that can be obtained by the tibial operation is again 5 cm, but the procedure can be repeated as the child grows.

Epiphyseal arrest. Limb-length discrepancy can also be treated by temporarily stopping growth at the lower femoral and upper tibial epiphyseal plates. This is achieved by placing staples across the growth plate, one prong being in the epiphysis and the other in the metaphysis. The advantage of this method is that the staples can be removed again at any time and growth then recommences provided that no damage has been done to the growth plate. The timing of stapling must be carefully planned using 'projected growth' charts in order to obtain the optimal result when growth is complete.

It is important to remember that the average adult can tolerate up to $2\frac{1}{2}$ cm of shortening of a lower limb without limping.

Scoliosis
Poliomyelitis usually causes the 'long C' type of paralytic curve. Procedures designed to balance muscle power have unfortunately proved ineffective. Treatment of the spinal curve is discussed in Chapter 16.

RECOMMENDATIONS FOR FURTHER READING

ILLINGWORTH, R. S. (1972) *The Development of the Infant and Young Child* (5th edn), Churchill Livingstone, London and Edinburgh.

RANG, M. (1966) Little's original description of cerebral palsy. In *Anthology of Orthopaedics*, pp. 48–52, E. & S. Livingstone, Edinburgh.

8 Infections of bone

Infections of bone may be acute (usually seen in children), subacute, or chronic. The subacute group is subdivided into a relapsing type, usually following an acute episode, and a primarily subacute type due to infection by an organism of limited virulence.

ACUTE OSTEOMYELITIS

Acute osteomyelitis (acute haemotogenous osteomyelitis) is a bacterial infection arising in the metaphyseal region of a bone.

Incidence
It is a disease of young people, usually affecting the bone before the epiphyseal lines have closed.

Bacteriology
Staphylococci are the commonest causative organisms (over 80 per cent). Others are pneumococci and streptococci. Rarely *Brucella* and typhoid organisms have been found.

Pathology
The long bones are usually involved. Infection reaches the metaphyseal region via the blood-stream from a septic focus elsewhere in the body, e.g. a boil or pharyngitis.

Once established the infection spreads in various directions: outwards to form a subperiosteal abscess; along the medullary cavity; directly into the synovial cavity of the neighbouring joint (especially if the metaphysis is intra-

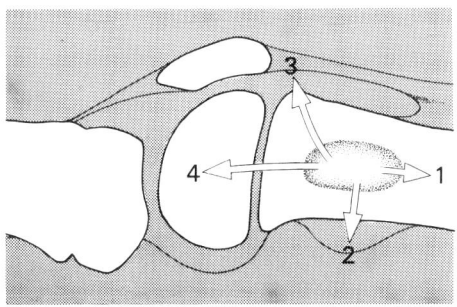

FIG. 8.1. The directions of spread of infection in acute osteomyelitis:
1) along the medullary canal
2) to the subperiosteal region
3) into the neighbouring joint
4) into and through the epiphysis

capsular); and often into and through the epiphysis (Fig. 8.1). In addition to the septic arthritis due to direct spread, effusions into joints near foci of osteomyelitis due to irritation of the synovium are common.

The formation of a subperiosteal abscess causes elevation of the periosteum and consequent cutting off of the blood-supply to the cortex of the bone. This ischaemia is increased if medullary spread of the infection affects the nutrient artery. The ischaemic area of bone undergoes necrosis and this area of dead bone is referred to as a 'sequestrum'. As the disease progresses, the elevated periosteum lays down layers of new bone which surround the sequestrated areas of bone. This new bone is referred to as an 'involucrum' and it may contain perforations known as 'cloacae' through which pus drains from the bone to the soft tissues of the limb.

During the early stages of the disease there is a septicaemia, which may endanger the life of the patient. Osteomyelitis carried a mortality rate of more than 50 per cent in the days before the introduction of antibiotics and is occasionally fatal even today.

Clinical picture
There is often a history of a knock or other minor injury in the affected area a few days prior to the onset of the illness. If the patient is seen early on in the disease, there may be very little in the way of physical signs: often no more than a little reddening and swelling over the affected bone. The bone is almost invariably tender to pressure. In babies the diagnosis may be difficult but usually the mother has noticed that the child is reluctant to use the limb.

As the condition progresses, the temperature rises and the patient becomes more toxic. Coma may supervene.

After a few days the presence of a subperiosteal abscess may become evident: the temperature becomes 'swinging' in nature and a fluctuant swelling is found in the affected area.

If the focus of infection is in a bone remote from the body surface, e.g. near the sciatic notch, local signs may be minimal.

Special investigations
1. *Blood culture.* A specimen of blood for culture should be taken as soon as the diagnosis is suspected and certainly before any antibiotic therapy is started as antibiotics will almost certainly destroy any chance of obtaining a positive result.
2. *White cell count.* There is usually a polymorphonuclear leucocytosis present but an overwhelming infection may depress the marrow and prevent or delay its onset.
3. *Erythrocyte sedimentation rate.* This is usually raised.
4. *Radiographs.* These are usually singularly uninformative in the early stages of the disease. The reason for this is that calcification has to be either increased or decreased for any change to be visible on X-ray, and this process takes about 10 days to occur. A good working rule is that 'the X-ray shows today what happened in the bone 2 weeks ago'. The earliest findings are mottling in the metaphyseal region and elevation of the periosteum.
5. *Bone scanning.* The rate of metabolism of bone may be studied by estimating the rate of uptake of radioactive strontium. In osteomyelitis, as would be expected, the rate of uptake is increased. The interesting point is that the

increased uptake continues long after there has been radiographic resolution of the lesion.

Treatment
As soon as the blood sample has been set up for culture, a course of antibiotic therapy is instituted. It is advisable to use a combination of two broad-spectrum antibiotics until the sensitivities of the organisms are known.

Careful observation of the patient at regular intervals is undertaken, special attention being directed to general condition, temperature, and pulse and progression of the local lesion. If the infection responds to the antibiotic therapy improvement is generally seen within 24 hours.

Surgical exploration of the lesion is indicated if:
(1) there is no response to antibiotic therapy;
(2) the general condition of the patient deteriorates;
(3) evidence of a subperiosteal or soft tissues abscess develops—a swinging temperature or fluctuation in the local lesion.

The bone is exposed, and if there is no collection of pus found under the periosteum, the cortex of the bone should be drilled. This usually reveals pus under pressure in the medullary cavity. A specimen is taken for bacteriological study. After taking steps to ensure that there is adequate drainage for any further pus which may form, the wound is closed.

Following exploration, there is usually an improvement in the patient's condition but it is important to continue the antibiotic therapy for some time after the temperature has returned to normal. A period of 6 weeks is considered the minimum.

In severe infections it is not unusual to find more than one focus of infection, the other site being either in another bone or a metastatic abscess in the lung, kidney, brain, or muscle. These foci should be treated on their merits.

Some surgeons prefer to explore the infected bone surgically as soon as the diagnosis is made. The advantages of this treatment is that the diagnosis is confirmed early in the course of the disease and a specimen for culture obtained. The disadvantage is that many patients respond to antibiotic therapy and do not require an operation.

Course and prognosis
Many cases respond satisfactorily to treatment. Occasionally the infection flares up again in the affected area and occasionally the patient returns with further infections in other bones. Death from osteomyelitis has become a rarity since the introduction of antibiotics.

SUBACUTE OSTEOMYELITIS

The commonest form of subacute osteomyelitis is the relapsing type. This follows an acute attack and suggests that the original infection has not completely responded to treatment.

A persistent abscess in the metaphyseal region of a bone is often referred to as a 'Brodie's abscess'.

Symptoms
The patient complains of attacks of pain, swelling, and redness either in the site of the primary infection or in some other focus. It is common for multiple sites to be affected at different times.

Signs
These are similar to those found in the acute type though not so marked. Toxaemia is not usually as severe.

Special investigations
1. Blood culture should be set up before antibiotic therapy is instituted.
2. White cell count is normally raised.
3. Erythrocyte sedimentation rate is usually raised.

Radiographs
If the recurrence of infection has occurred in a previously affected part of the bone, radiographs will show a loss of normal architecture, and, in addition, a sequestrum may be found. This shows as a dense area or fragment of bone usually surrounded by less dense bone.

Course
Untreated, the infection leads to abscess and sinus formation. If sinuses have been present for several years, the possibility of amyloidosis should be considered.

Treatment
Most recurrent flares respond to a course of the relevant antibiotics. If a sequestrum is present it is unlikely that the infection will settle until the sequestrum is removed.

Typhoid osteomyelitis
Bone infection by *Salmonella typhi* is rare but does occur in countries where typhoid fever is not as well controlled as it is here in Britain.

Brucellosis
The possibility of *Brucella* infection should be considered in any subacute osteomyelitis especially if occurring in a patient associated with agricultural activities.

CHRONIC OSTEOMYELITIS—TUBERCULOSIS OF BONE

The commonest and most important type of chronic infection of bone is that due to tuberculosis. Within the last 20 years the number of cases of bone tuberculosis has greatly diminished and it has almost disappeared completely. However, the last few years has seen the reappearance of occasional cases—both in the indigenous population and, to a greater extent, in immigrants.

Cause
The *Mycobacterium tuberculosis* reaches the bone via the blood-stream. The initial site of infection, e.g. the lung, may still be active or—more commonly—has healed by the time the skeletal focus is discovered. The bone lesion may be found close to a joint in association with tuberculous arthritis or may have no connection with a joint lesion, e.g. in the greater trochanter or vertebral body.

Infections of the vertebral column and of the finger (TB dactylitis) deserve individual description.

Spinal tuberculosis

Pathology
The infection usually starts within the body of a vertebra. As area of inflamation is set up with surrounding hyperaemia and thinning of bone. Softening of the bone causes collapse and the intervertebral discs become displaced into the bodies of the vertebrae. Abscess formation on either side of the spine is common (Fig. 8.2).

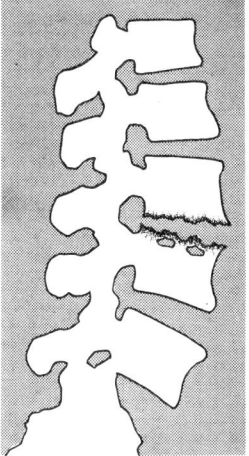

FIG. 8.2. Radiographic tracing of a case of tuberculousis of the fourth lnmbar vertebra.

Special investigations
1. Radiographs may show a paraspinal abscess, loss of bone density, collapse of vertebral bodies, and loss of disc space.
2. Full blood count may show lymphocytosis.
3. Microscopical examination of the sputum may show the presence of tuberculous bacilli (Zeil–Nielsen stain) and culture of the sputum may reveal tubercle bacilli.

Treatment
The traditional treatment for spinal tuberculosis was to immobilize the patient on a plaster bed and administer antituberculous drugs—streptomycin, *p*-aminosalicylic acid (PAS) and isonicotinic acid hydrazide (INAH). The response to treatment was gauged by estimating the erythrocyte sedimentation rate and by radiography. The period of immobilization varied greatly but was seldom less than 6–12 months.

This method is still in use, but controlled trials have suggested that bed rest may not be essential. Some patients therefore are treated by immobilizing the spine in a support, administering antituberculous drugs, and allowing the patient to lead an active life. A periodic check is carried out, the ESR being estimated and radiographs taken.

Care must be taken to identify early any side effects of the drug therapy. PAS and INAH tend to cause nausea. Streptomycin affects the eighth cranial nerve and may cause deafness. Side effects are also caused by several new antituberculous drugs on the market: rifampicin can cause mild liver toxicity and bone marrow depression; ethambutol can cause nausea and vomiting; and ethionamide can cause nausea and vomiting and occasional retrobulbar neuritis.

The above methods of treatment may be called conservative. The Hong Kong school are the main proponents of operative treatment: they recommend removal of diseased vertebral bodies and other tissue and replacement with bone grafts—antituberculous drugs are given in addition. The results in their series compare very favourably with those of the conservative school.

Complications
1. Generalized miliary tuberculosis, which may be fatal.
2. Paraplegia, either of early onset due to extension of the abscess into the spinal canal, or late onset due to deformity of the spine with subsequent traction on the spinal cord.

Sequela. A kyphotic deformity, usually of the knuckle type, is often seen in the disease of the thoracic region.

Tuberculous dactylitis
This usually occurs in the metacarpal or phalanx of a finger.

Clinical features
The metacarpal region or part of finger is warm, tender, and thickened.

Radiographs
These show a characteristic loss of the normal outline. The shaft of the bone is widened and the whole bone has a coarse, foamy appearance.

Treatment
Rest, antituberculous drugs, and, later, currettage of bone, if the infection does not subside on conservative treatment.

RECOMMENDATIONS FOR FURTHER READING

BLOCKEY, N. J. and WATSON, J. T. (1970) Acute osteomyelitis in children, *J. Bone Jt Surg.* **52B**, 77–87.

NICHOLSON, R. A. (1974) Twenty years of bone and joint tuberculosis in Bradford, *J. Bone Jt Surg.* **56B**, 760–5.

WILKINSON, M. C. (1969) Tuberculosis of the spine treated by chemotherapy and operative debridement, *J. Bone Jt Surg.* **51A**, 1331–42.

9 Infections of joints

Bacterial infection of joints may be acute or chronic. Acute infections may be caused by blood-borne bacteria or by direct inoculation during trauma. As mentioned in the chapter on osteomyelitis, it is important to appreciate that the infection of the joint may be secondary to infection of a neighbouring bone.

ACUTE SEPTIC ARTHRITIS

Since acute septic arthritis presents such a different clinical picture in the very young and the old, these two conditions will be described separately.

Acute septic arthritis in children

Cause
This usually follows penetrating wounds of joint but blood-spread infections do occur. Very often what was thought to be a primary septic arthritis later turns out to have been an osteomyelitis of a neighbouring bone, the delay in onset of radiological findings contributing to the deception.

Symptoms
Acute pain on any movement of the joint. The patient is often pyrexial and toxic.

Signs
The joint is swollen and tender and attempted movement in any direction is painful. If the joint is superficial, e.g. the knee, it may be felt to be warm and the overlying skin may be red.

Special investigations
There is a polymorphonuclear leucocytosis and the erythrocyte sedimentation rate is raised. Aspiration of the joint yields pus or infected synovial fluid which should be cultured bacteriologically and the antibiotic sensitivity of the causative organism assessed.

Radiographs. The radiological joint space may be increased due to the presence of fluid in the joint.

Treatment
 1. Rest: the limb is splinted or, in the case of the hip, traction is applied.
 2. Antibiotics are administered. If the causative organism and its sensitivity are known the relevant antibiotic(s) are given; if not, a broad-spectrum antibiotic is given. It is important not to commence antibiotic treatment until an aspiration specimen and a blood sample has been taken for culture.

48 Orthopaedics for Undergraduates

3. Aspiration or operative drainage may be necessary for gross pyoarthroses or for those not responding to the conservative measures described above. Some surgeons institute continuous perfusion of the joint cavity with an antibiotic solution. This is not often required.

4. It should be stressed that the hip is a very difficult joint to assess and it is my practice to explore the hip if there is any suggestion of intra-articular infection.

Results. In children resolution is the rule except in the case of suppurative arthritis of the hip in infancy, which may cause necrosis of the capital epiphysis of the femur.

Acute septic arthritis in adults
Although the bacteriology and pathology of adult cases may be the same as in those occurring in children, the clinical presentation may be very different—the picture is much less acute and the surgeon may be lulled into a false sense of security. This may lead to delay in operative drainage until marked destruction of joint and neighbouring bone have occurred.

Often the only indications of the disease are malaise, pyrexia, and aching in the joint with some spasm of associated muscles on moving the joint. It may be tender to palpation. Diagnostic aspiration or exploration is recommended if any doubt exists as to the diagnosis.

Treatment
This follows the same lines as in the case of children—the administration of the appropriate antibiotics and aspiration or drainage if there is not a satisfactory response to conservative treatment. In the case of the hip joint, drainage should be undertaken sooner rather than later since the deep position of the joint makes assessment more difficult and may cause a delay in diagnosis.

Results. Unlike the situation in children, septic arthritis in adults usually causes articular cartilage damage with resultant joint stiffness and pain and occasionally complete bony fusion of the joint.

CHRONIC INFECTIVE ARTHRITIS

The common organism causing chronic infective arthritis is *M. tuberculosis*, as in the case of chronic osteomyelitis.

Up to the time of the Second World War, TB arthritis was very common. Pasteurization of milk has virtually eliminated infection by the bovine type of bacillus, and the introduction of antituberculous drugs—streptomycin, *p*-aminosalicylic acid, and isonicotinic acid hydrazide—has drastically reduced the number of cases seen. The disease is, however, relatively common in the immigrant population.

Pathology
The joint infection is virtually never the primary site of disease. The current belief is that the patient has had a previous infection—probably in the lung—which has been brought under control but never completely eradicated. Some bacteria later escape from the affected lymph nodes, perhaps during a period of intercurrent illness, circulate in the blood-stream, and finally settle in the joint.

Infection starts either in the synovium (tubercular synovitis) or in the bone adjacent to the joint, subsequently entering it by direct spread. The synovium becomes inflamed and thickened and effusions occur into the joint. If the disease progresses, the articular cartilage becomes ulcerated and the underlying bone destroyed. Abscesses may occur which track towards the skin surface, discharge, and form sinuses. Sinuses allow bacteria other than *M. tuberculosis* to enter the joint and secondary infection supervenes.

If the articular cartilage is destroyed, healing is by fibrosis with the formation of a fibrous ankylosis. If secondary infection has supervened, healing by bone fusion may occur (bony ankylosis).

Symptoms
The patient is usually a child or young adult. There may be no history of symptoms attributable to the primary infection. Pain in the affected joint may be slight or severe—characteristically attacks of pain come on at night, waking the patient from sleep as the joint is moved. General malaise, lassitude, and loss of weight are common.

Signs
Early stages. The large joints—hip, knee, ankle, and elbow—are the commonest affected. The joint may be slightly swollen and synovial thickening may be palpable. Effusions are common. Muscle wasting is common even in early cases. This is seen, for example, in the quadriceps muscle in knee infections.

Spasm of the muscles acting on the joint is found when the joint is moved suddenly. Restriction in the range of movement with pain at the extremes of movement are common.

Late stages. Fibrous ankylosis either abolishes all movement of the joint or allows only a 'jog' of movement to occur. In bony ankylosis, of course, there is no movement. Muscle wasting may be extreme. Sinuses may be present and the joint may be swollen because of swelling of the synovium and brawny oedema of the subcutaneous tissues.

Sinuses or the scars of healed sinuses are seen. In the case of knee and hip infections, it is important to look for sinuses or their scars on the posterior aspect of the joint.

Radiographs
In the early stages there may be soft tissue shadows indicative of synovial swelling. The hyperaemia leads to decalcification of bone so that the density of the bones forming the joint is diminished. A focus of infection in a neighbouring bone may be visible.

In the later stages, loss of joint space and destruction of subchondral bone becomes evident.

After some years, bony ankylosis leads to complete loss of evidence that a joint has ever been present: the bony trabelculae are continuous across the area of the previous joint space.

Special investigations
1. The white cell count is elevated and there is often a relative lymphocytosis.
2. The erythrocyte sedimentation rate is elevated—this test is commonly used in monitoring the response of a patient under treatment: it provides a sensitive index of the progression of the disease.

3. The Mantoux test may be useful in cases in which the diagnosis is in doubt.
4. Aspiration of effusions—direct examination may show the presence of acid-fast bacilli but this is rare. Guinea-pig inoculation testing is more likely to give positive results.

Treatment
1. Rest is important and should be continued until the disease is quiescent.
2. Antituberculous drugs are essential and should be used in combinations of two or three given simultaneously. The use of one drug on its own rapidly leads to the development of resistance.
3. Surgical excision of all infected tissue is advocated by some schools and certainly has a place in the treatment of the more advanced case.
4. In late cases with joint destruction, the limb should be immobilized in optimum position for the inevitable ankylosis to occur.
5. After the disease has become quiescent, rehabilitation of the patient and the diseased joint is commenced.

Results
If treatment is started before the articular cartilage has been destroyed, a return to a normal or near-normal joint can be expected. If the cartilage has been destroyed a stiff joint will result. The infective lesion can usually be brought under control.

Occasionally, the infection becomes widespread and involves other systems besides the skeletal system. Overwhelming infections do still occur occasionally—with fatal results.

RECOMMENDATIONS FOR FURTHER READING

GRIFFITHS, D. L., SEDDON, H. J., and ROAF, R. (1956) *Potts' Paraplegia*, Oxford University Press, London.

RANG, M. (1966) Tom Smith's arthritis, original description. In *Anthology of Orthopaedics*, pp. 16-17, E. & S. Livingstone, Edinburgh.

WILKINSON, M. C. (1969) Tuberculosis of the hip and knee treated by chemotherapy, synovectomy and debridement, *J. Bone Jt Surg.* **51A**, 1343-59.

10 Degenerative arthrosis

Wearing out of joints—or degenerative arthrosis—is one of the commonest conditions encountered in orthopaedics. Two main types exist.
1. *Primary osteoarthrosis.* In this type there is no known cause for the degeneration.
2. *Secondary osteoarthrosis.* In this type there has been previous destruction of articular cartilage or deformation of the joint surfaces.

Although it is by no means confined to them, degenerative arthritis causes most signs and symptoms when it affects the weight-bearing joints—the hips, the knees, and the ankles.

Other joints commonly affected are the elbow joints, the wrist joints, and the carpo-metacarpal joints of the thumbs. It may also occur in the metacarpo-phalangeal and interphalangeal joints of the fingers if these have been affected previously by rheumatoid disease.

It is only in recent years that the term osteoarthrosis has been in common use. Prior to this degeneration of joints was called 'osteoarthritis'—a term still often heard today.

Causes
The secondary type may follow:
1. Previous intra-articular fractures and injuries to the articular cartilage.
2. Septic arthritis.
3. Rheumatoid arthritis.
4. Osteochondritis, e.g. Perthes' or Freiberg's disease.
5. Osteochondritis dissecans, in which an area of articular cartilage and underlying bone undergoes necrosis and separates from the surrounding bone.
6. Deformities of the limb which upset the mechanics of the joint.

In the primary type the cause is unknown.

Clinical features
Three main symptoms are usually mentioned.

Pain
This is felt in the region of the joint and along the muscles acting on the joint. Characteristically, the pain is worse on using the joint after resting. In the later stages it becomes continuous and may interfere with sleep. Occasionally a degenerative hip may cause pain which is referred to the medial side of the knee.

Stiffness
A large proportion of the range of movement of a joint may be lost before

the patient notices any restriction. Characteristically the restriction of hip joint movement is not noticed until the patient encounters difficulty with putting on his shoes and socks.

Deformity
With progressive reduction in the range of movement of the joint, the limb tends to rest in a deformed position. Finally the joint will become stiff in this position, e.g. the hip usually adopts the position of flexion, adduction, and external rotation. The adduction deformity forces the patient to elevate the pelvis on the arthritic side when walking in order to keep his legs from hitting together and this leads to the common belief by the patient that his affected leg is shorter than the sound one.

Signs
The physical signs confirm the symptoms:

Pain
Discomfort on moving the joint is common, especially at the extremes of the range.

Stiffness
Restriction in range of one or more of the movements of the joint is usually found.

Deformity
The joint may be held in a deformed position, e.g. hip flexed, adducted, and externally rotated or the deformity which has predisposed to the degenerative change may be seen, e.g. genu varum causing medial compartment changes in the knee.

Radiographs
There are four main characteristic findings which may be present:

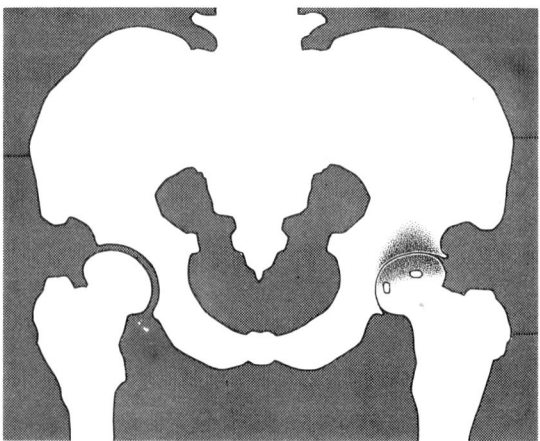

FIG. 10.1. The radiographic changes of degenerative arthrosis of the left hip.

Loss of the radiological joint space
This space on the radiograph represents that part of the joint which consists mainly of articular cartilage and to a lesser extent other intra-articular soft tissue, e.g. menisci. Diminution of this space implies that the articular cartilage has been eroded (Fig. 10.1).

Sclerosis (increased density)
There is sclerosis of the bone adjacent to the articular surfaces.

Osteophytes
These are areas of heaped up new bone at the margins of the articular surfaces.

Cysts
These occur in the bone adjacent to the articular surfaces.

Course and prognosis
Untreated, the disease runs a progressive course characterized by remissions and relapses. There is a great variation in the degree of severity of symptoms and signs in different patients.

Treatment

Conservative treatment
This is often successful in relieving pain (the commonest symptom causing the patient to attend hospital) and in increasing the range of movement in the affected joint.

Pain relief is afforded by analgesics, e.g. phenylbutazone, by reducing the load on the joint by the use of a walking-stick, and by splintage of the affected joint. Heat applied locally to the joint either as radiant heat or as short-wave diathermy is specific for pain relief in osteoarthritis.

Mobilizing exercises, which should be active, i.e. done by the patient's own muscles and within the limits of discomfort, help to retain and, in some cases, increase the range of movement.

Operative treatment
This is indicated if conservative measures have failed. Three main operations are done.
1. *Arthrodesis.* In this operation the joint is stiffened permanently. This gives complete relief of pain but throws an increased strain on the other joints in the area. For this reason it is usually confined to younger patients before the adaptability of the other joints has been affected. It is most often used in the hip, knee, wrist, and ankle.
2. *Osteotomy.* It has been found that the pain of osteoarthritis can usually be relieved by cutting across the bone distal to the arthritic joint and then allowing it to unite in a slightly altered position. This also affords an opportunity for correcting any deformity which may be present. Internal or external fixation of the 'fractured' bone is then used until it has united (Fig. 10.2).

Pain relief is the almost invariable rule after osteotomy. The prognosis for movement range is not so predictable.
3. *Arthroplasty.* This implies the making of a new joint and there are several methods by which this can be done.
    (a) One or both of the articular surfaces of the bones forming the joint may be excised and the resultant gap allowed to fill with fibrous tissue.

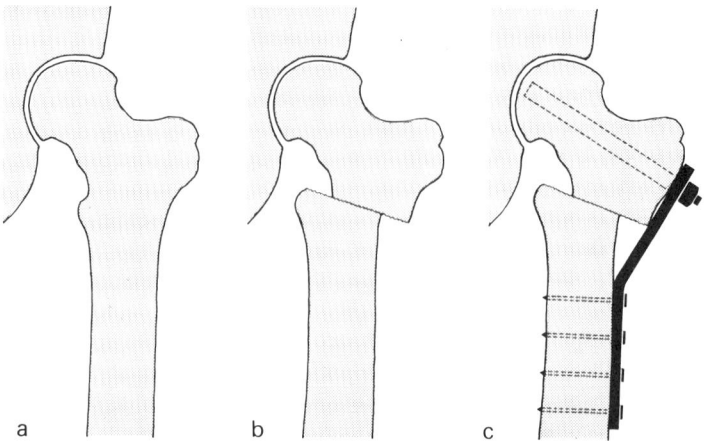

FIG. 10.2. Displacement osteotomy of McMurray. (a) Preoperative position. (b) Level of osteotomy. (c) Application of internal fixation.

(b) One of both bony components of the joint may be excised and replaced by a metal or plastic substitute. Many joints are successfully treated in this way, the commonest being the knee (Shier's hinge or other two-part prostheses) and the hip (Charnley, McKee–Farrar, or Ring prostheses; see Fig. 10.3).

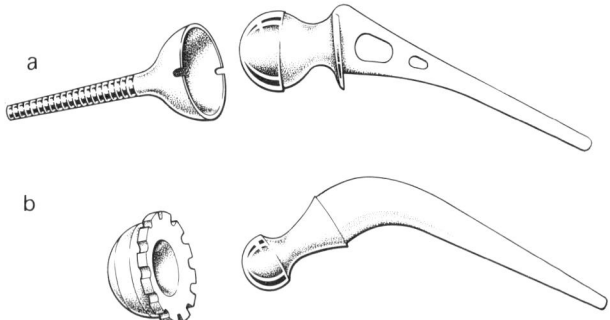

FIG. 10.3. (a) The Ring (metal-to-metal) hip replacement prosthesis. (b) The Charnley (metal-to-plastic) hip replacement prosthesis.

Results. Arthrodesis and osteotomy can generally be relied on to relieve pain. In arthrodesis all movement is lost and in osteotomy the range of movement may be increased or decreased. Arthroplasty without replacement results in some instability of the joint and with replacement usually gives a very satisfactory result. It is, as yet, too early to assess the long-term results of total joint replacement.

RECOMMENDATIONS FOR FURTHER READING

BULLOUGH, P. and GOODFELLOW, J. (1968) The significance of the fine structure of articular cartilage, *J. Bone Jt Surg.* **50B**, 852–7.

11 Generalized conditions of bone

There are many conditions which tend to affect several bones or the skeleton as a whole. This chapter consists of a summary of the more important conditions which you are likely to encounter: it does not claim to be a complete survey. For convenience we have divided the conditions into groups according to their aetiology:
 (1) generalized conditions of congenital origin;
 (2) generalized conditions due to hormonal dysfunction;
 (3) generalized conditions due to dietary and metabolic causes;
 (4) generalized conditions of unknown aetiology.

GENERALIZED CONDITIONS OF BONE OF CONGENITAL ORIGIN

Osteogenesis imperfecta (fragilitas ossium)
This is a relatively rare condition characterized by abnormal fragility or brittleness of bone.

Cause
An inherited condition passed on as a dominant gene with no sex predilection.

Types
1. *Foetal type.* In this condition intra-uterine fractures occur. Ossification of the skull is delayed and stillbirth is common.
2. *Infantile type.* This is a less severe form. Fractures are less numerous, but the prognosis for life is still very limited.
3. *Adolescent type (osteogenesis imperfecta tarda).* In this type the child is normal at birth, but the tendency to fractures later becomes apparent. Fractures become less common as the child gets older.

Signs
The child is usually dwarfed. The head is globular in shape: the frontal bones may be bossed. Kyphosis and scoliosis are common and the limbs show gross deformities due both to deficient growth and previous fractures. Hypermobility of the joints is also seen.

Blue sclerae are common. This appearance is due to the dark choroid showing through an abnormally translucent sclera. Deafness is present in more than 50 per cent of cases.

Radiographs
The skull shows the presence of Wormian bones (irregular islands of ossifica-

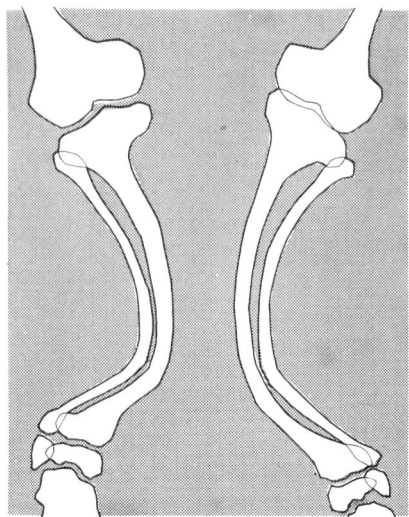

FIG. 11.1. Osteogenesis imperfecta. The radiographic appearance of the leg bones following multiple fractures.

tion), a high dome, and marked radiotranslucency. The pelvis may be trefoil in shape and the limb bones show multiple old fractures (Fig. 11.1).

Pathology
Bones show absence of normal cortex, and histology reveals areas of immature and unorganized bone.

Treatment
The child should be protected from injury. Deformities may be corrected by osteotomy or osteoclasis. Bizarre deformities of long bones are occasionally corrected by multiple osteotomies and insertion of an intramedullary rod. Fracture healing is excellent.

Prognosis
The prognosis for life in all severe cases is poor. The child usually succumbs to pulmonary infections.

Diaphyseal aclasia (multiple exostosis)
This is a relatively common condition characterized by failure of moulding of the metaphyseal region of long bones and the presence of exostoses arising from the metaphysis. It is really more of a metaphyseal than diaphyseal affection.

Cause
This is an inherited condition commoner in males than in females.

Pathology
Periosteal moulding of the metaphyseal region is lost. Small islands of carti-

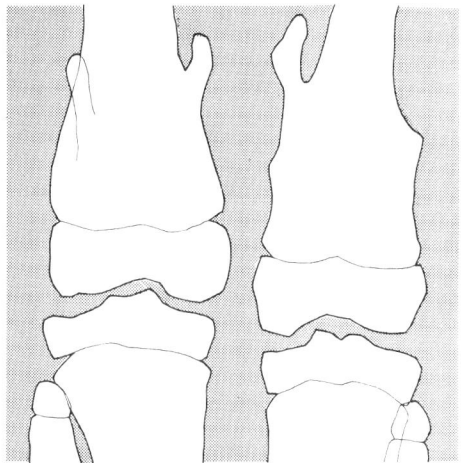

FIG. 11.2. Radiographic appearance of exostoses in the knee regions in a case of diaphyseal aclasia.

lage become separated from the main bone and give rise to slender cartilage capped exostoses. The metaphysis is also broader than normal. The main bones affected are the femur, tibia, fibula, ulna, radius, and humerus.

Symptoms

The patient usually attends hospital because the swellings in the regions of the knees, ankles, or shoulders have been noticed. Occasionally tendons may 'flick' over the exostoses causing discomfort and interference with muscle action.

Signs

Bony swellings are palpable near the joints. These children tend to be short in stature.

Radiographs

These show widening of the metaphysis and the exostoses arising from the metaphysis and growing towards the centre of the diaphysis, i.e. away from the neighbouring joint (Fig. 11.2).

Treatment

Excision of troublesome exostoses is indicated.

Prognosis

Malignant degeneration rarely occurs in these tumours. In the absence of this, life expectancy is normal.

Dyschondroplasia (multiple enchondromata; Ollier's disease)

An hereditary disease, without sex predilection, dyschondroplasia is characterized by multiple areas of cartilage within the bones of the pelvis, limbs, hands, and feet.

Pathology
The bones show lack of organization at the metaphyseal regions, the defects being within the bone rather than protruding from it. Usually one bone or one limb alone is affected.

Signs
Unequal growth of limbs is usually the first sign. Swellings at the metaphyseal regions of long bones or in the hands are common. Deformities due to interference with growth later supervene.

Radiographs
These show areas of translucency and spots of increased calcification in the metaphyses of long bones and in the phalanges, metacarpals, and metatarsals. Radiating lines of translucency may be seen in the ilium.

Treatment
Operative correction of deformities may be necessary, but should if possible be delayed until skeletal maturity.

Prognosis
Prognosis for life is good, although occasionally sarcomatous change occurs.

Achondroplasia
The condition is characterized by dwarfing: a virtually normal-sized trunk with short limbs and a large head. Intelligence and muscle power are normal or above average.

Cause
Hereditary defect of pre-bone cartilage.

Pathology
The normal column formation of cartilage cells during bone growth does not occur. Periosteal bone formation is normal. The resulting bone is therefore short, but thick and strong. Membranous bone is not affected.

Signs
At birth the child is found to have a normal trunk and short limbs; the fingers are all the same length; there is a characteristic depression at the root of the nose; and the head is large.

As the child develops, the vault of the skull (membrane bone) increases in size, but the base of skull and face (cartilage bone) do not develop to the same extent. The shortness of the limbs is more marked in the proximal segments (thigh or arm) and bow-leg is characteristic, as is increased lumbar lordosis. These individuals are commonly seen as circus dwarfs.

Radiographs
These show shortened bones with wide metaphyses.

Treatment
Excessive bowing may require operative correction.

Prognosis
These individuals have a normal life expectancy.

Generalized conditions of bone 59

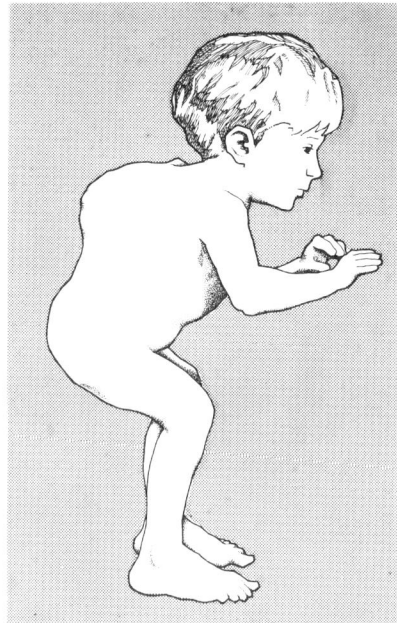

FIG. 11.3. Child suffering from osteochondrodystrophy (Morquio–Brailsford type).

Osteochondrodystrophy

This condition was thought previously to be a single entity, but the discovery of varying types of mucopolysaccharide and other metabolic abnormalities has led to the establishment of a dozen or more subdivisions of it. The most important features of the group as a whole will be described.

Pathology

Growth of pre-bone cartilage and subsequent ossification are both defective. The relative rate of growth of bones does not conform to the normal pattern. Osteochondritic lesions similar to those seen in Perthes' disease may occur in the weight-bearing joints.

Vertebral bodies show variations in shape characteristic of the various types of disease, e.g. a flattened body with a central tongue is seen in the Morquio–Brailsford variety (Fig. 11.3). Kyphosis is common.

Signs

The child appears normal at birth but with subsequent growth develops shortening of the neck, kyphosis of the lumbar spine, and flexion deformities of the knees and hips resulting in the characteristic crouched posture which, if markedly developed, prevents the child from standing.

Radiographs

These may show cavernous acetabula, flattened vertebrae, short thick lower limb bones, overgrowth of the radius, and kyphosis.

It must be emphasized that there are variations in this condition and that not all of these features are found in every case.

Treatment
There is no specific treatment for the underlying metabolic congenital defect. The various deformities may require operative correction.

Prognosis
There is a normal life expectancy in this condition.

Craniocleidodysostosis
An inherited condition with deficient development of membrane bone, particularly clavicles and vault of skull.

Signs
The face is flat, the skull globular, the clavicles may be completely or partly absent so that the shoulders may be brought in contact with each other across the chest.
The perineum may be wide due to coxa vara.

Radiographs
These show the presence of a metopic (midline) suture in the frontal bone: the deficient clavicles; the coxa vara; and occasionally widening of the symphysis pubis.

Treatment
The coxa vara may require operative treatment if severe.

Prognosis
Life expectancy is normal.

Osteopetrosis (marble bones)
A rare familiar condition characterized by brittle bones which on X-ray are shown to be excessively dense: no differentiation into cortex and medulla is discernible. In addition to increased brittleness, the condition causes depression of marrow function and compression of cranial nerves within the base of the skull. Treatment is symptomatic.

GENERALIZED CONDITIONS OF BONE DUE TO HORMONAL DYSFUNCTION

There are two clinical conditions to be discussed in this group: hypothyroidism and hyperparathyroidism.

Hypothyroidism
Hyposecretion of thyroid hormone may occur at any age and, in adults, gives rise to the condition of myxoedema. Patients suffering from this condition usually present in the medical clinics and there are no characteristic orthopaedic problems.

In infancy and childhood, however, hypothyroidism causes cretinism and the patient may well appear in the orthopaedic department. The child may be seen because of delay in walking or because of bow-legs or because its growth is stunted. As the child grows the condition becomes more apparent but it is important to diagnose these children as early as possible so that substitution therapy may be started. Often the earliest clue is the late appearance of secondary ossific centres in the epiphyses (e.g. of the lower femur or upper tibia). Indeed, the diagnosis is often suggested by the radiologist reporting on films taken for other conditions.

Investigation and treatment is usually carried out by paediatricians.

Hyperparathyroidism

The primary effect of the parathyroid hormone is to increase the excretion of phosphates in the urine. This has a secondary effect of raising the serum calcium. The rise in the serum calcium is brought about by reabsorption of calcium from the skeleton into the blood. In hyperparathyroidism there is a rise in the serum calcium, a drop in the serum phosphate, and an increased secretion of phosphorus in the urine. All three of these should be present before a confident diagnosis of hyperparathyroidism is made. There is a lot of truth, therefore, in the remark made by one of the tutors at the Royal College of Surgeons that hyperparathyroidism is the condition in which 'the patient gradually passes his skeleton in his urine'.

Clinical picture
Hypercalcaemia may cause nausea, vomiting, weight loss, abdominal pain, and muscular weakness.

Radiological changes
There is at first a generalized diminution in bone density. The resorption of bone from around the teeth (lamina dura) is characteristic. Later on in the disease, areas of bone resorption in the form of cysts may be found. Resorption is also seen in the subperiosteal layers of the phalanges of the fingers. Granular mottling of the calvarium may be seen on the skull radiograph. There are other manifestations of hypercalcaemia seen on radiography, e.g. metastatic calcification, renal nephrocalcinosis, and renal stones.

In 1891 von Recklinghausen described three cases of 'generalized osteitis fibrosa cystica'. This cystic degeneration of bone is seen in hyperparathyroidism. It is interesting to note that two of the three cases he described were later found to be suffering from polyostotic fibrous dysplasia.

The cystic areas in bone usually imply that the disease is of long standing, and in the past were referred to as 'brown tumours'—a misnomer because the swelling is neither brown (it is red) nor is it a tumour. It is in fact a cystic resorption of bone in this area. The radiological appearance of these cystic areas may be similar to the giant-cell tumour and diagnosis may be a problem if a single cystic area is encountered.

Histologically the differentiation is not very difficult. The large cells in hyperparathyroidism are macrophages as against giant cells in giant cell tumours, and the stroma in hyperparathyroidism is fibrous rather than spindle cell.

Treatment
The treatment is directed to the parathyroid glands, which are explored and any tumour or hyperplastic area removed. This operation is, of course, usually carried out by general surgeons.

GENERALIZED CONDITIONS OF BONE DUE TO DIETARY AND METABOLIC CAUSES

Three conditions will be described under this heading—dietary rickets, renal rickets, and osteomalacia.

Dietary rickets

Dietary rickets causes softening of bone with resultant bending. It is very rarely seen today because the importance of dietary calcium and vitamin D, and of sunlight, are appreciated. In the early years of the century, on the other hand, a great deal of the orthopaedic surgeons' work was concerned with the correction of rachitic deformities and operation lists usually contained two or three corrective osteotomies or osteoclases (fracturing of bones) for such deformities.

In present-day practice the condition is occasionally seen in dark-skinned immigrant children.

Clinical presentation
The child presents with swellings in the vicinity of joints which may be tender. Deformity of weight-bearing bones is rare today but classically used to affect the lower third of the tibiae. Some inward bending of the lower ribs due to softening and deformation due to the pull of the diaphragm may be seen (Harrison's sulci).

Radiographs
These show expansion and fuzziness of the metaphyseal regions so that the diaphysis appears to expand into the shape of the trumpet mouth at the metaphysis (Fig. 11.4). The anterior ends of the ribs may also be expanded giving rise to the clinical swellings at the costo-chondral junctions (rickety rosary).

Treatment
Improvement of diet and supplements of vitamin D and calcium are indicated. Correction of deformity is very rarely necessary in contemporary practice.

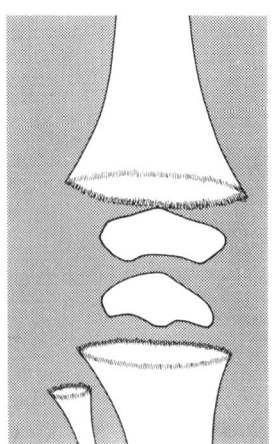

FIG. 11.4. Radiograph of the knee of a child suffering from rickets.

Renal rickets

The skeletal changes of rickets, or osteomalacia if the patient is adult, may be seen in patients whose diet is not deficient in vitamin D but who are suffering from renal disease. The coexistence of bone changes and renal disease was first reported by Lucas in 1883 and since then many detailed syndromes have been reported. It is now generally accepted that the signs of rickets may be found in two types of kidney diseases: chronic glomerulonephritis; and the numerous varieties of tubular resorption defects. Some of these varieties respond to massive doses of vitamin D and others do not and are referred to as vitamin D resistant rickets.

Treatment is directed to the underlying renal lesion.

Osteomalacia

Defective bone formation due to lack of essential materials, in adults, is referred to as osteomalacia. Although deficient intake may cause osteomalacia most cases seen today are due to deficient absorption. It is seen in the post-gastrectomy syndrome and any condition associated with intestinal 'hurry' or malabsorption, e.g. Crohn's disease or ulcerative colitis.

The investigation of these cases is usually undertaken in metabolic units and the orthopaedic surgeon is usually only concerned with the original diagnosis. These patients may present with pathological fractures and radiographs of the fractures may show areas of loss of bone substance in other bones or other parts of the same bone. These are called 'Looser's zones' or pseudo-fractures and are particularly common in the ribs and pubic rami. The serum alkaline phosphatase is almost invariably raised.

Biopsy of bone in these cases shows that mineralization of the trabeculae is deficient and that the seam of unossified osteoid on the surface of the trabecula is widened. The commonly used site for biopsy is the iliac crest.

Once the fracture has been treated and the diagnosis of osteomalacia made, the elucidation of the cause and its correction is carried out in the Metabolic Unit because of its special facilities for critical metabolic balance studies.

GENERALIZED CONDITIONS OF BONE OF UNKNOWN AETIOLOGY

Three conditions will be described under this heading: Paget's disease; osteoporosis; and fibrous dysplasia of bone.

Paget's disease

This is a condition of the middle-aged and the elderly, characterized by deformity of bones, particularly the long bones. Its other name is osteitis deformans.

The disease may affect one or many bones. The affected bone becomes larger than normal and on radiography the texture of the bone becomes more coarse. The progress of the changes down the shaft of a long bone may be studied by serial radiography: the advancing edge of the condition is characteristically V-shaped. It is believed that the condition results from a breakdown of the normal bone-deposition/bone-resorption balance.

Two stages of the disease are described. In the first the bone is hyperaemic and soft. At this stage the characteristic bowing occurs. In the second or chronic phase the bone becomes increasingly hard. Unfortunately it also becomes brittle and fractures may occur. These are often of the 'stress' type and therefore are undisplaced.

Clinical features
The patient may complain of pain in the early stages but very often the condition is painless and the patient seeks advice because of the deformity which is due to bowing of the femur or tibia.

This bowing may be either lateral or anterior. The limb feels warm in the earlier stages. Pain coming on late in the condition suggests that either a stress fracture has occurred or that malignant change (to osteosarcoma) has supervened.

The bones most commonly affected are the long bones of the lower limbs, the pelvis, the lumbar vertebra, and the skull.

Paget's disease of the pelvis seldom gives rise to pain unless the acetabulum is involved, in which case degenerative arthrosis may be superimposed. The pelvis may be softened and deformed into the trefoil shape (as in osteogenesis imperfecta).

Skull involvement may be preceded by a large area of osteoporosis (osteoporosis circumscripta) and when it spreads to involve the whole skull causes increase in thickness of the calvarium with consequent increase in the cranial circumference, the patient characteristically requiring a larger hat each year. Involvement of the base of the skull may cause compression of cranial nerves and deafness is not uncommon.

Involvement of the spine is usually localized to a single vertebral body, characteristically in the lumbar region. Radiographs show a single dense vertebral body. Care must be taken to exclude the other causes of this finding namely metastases from a prostatic carcinoma or, more rarely, a carcinoma of the breast.

Special investigations
Characteristically the serum alkaline phosphatase, the urinary calcium, and hydroxyproline excretion are all raised. The blood chemistry is normal in other respects.

Treatment
Until recently the treatment of Paget's disease was confined to pain relief, the correction of deformities, and the management of the three complications—pathological fractures, high-output cardiac failure, and malignant degeneration. In 1963 the hormone calcitonin was discovered. This has an effect approximately opposite to that of parathyroid hormone, namely it promotes the deposition of calcium in bone. It is the local practice to use calcitonin in cases of Paget's disease in which a joint is involved and to use another drug—fluoride—which promotes calcium deposition in bone for those cases involving bone only. The efficacy of treatment is gauged by monitoring the urinary output of calcium and hydroxyproline. Initial results are encouraging.

Malignant change in Paget's disease
Classically, malignant degeneration in a bone affected by Paget's disease is associated with swelling, pain, warmth, and tenderness. The diagnosis of malignant change may be extremely difficult in some cases, especially if the bone is deeply placed, e.g. the ischium.

Radiographs may show an area of disorganization and marked new bone formation but more often merely show a suspicious area. In these cases the serum alkaline phosphase may not be raised to a higher figure than that due to the Paget's disease. Some help may be obtained from the level of urinary hydroxyproline, but biopsy may have to be a last resort.

If there has been recent trauma to the suspect area, particularly if there has been a fracture, the histologist may be unable to distinguish reaction from malignant change and the decision has to be made entirely on clinical grounds.

Osteoporosis

It is intended to discuss under this heading the idiopathic type of generalized osteoporosis. This should not be confused with the localized type of osteoporosis which accompanies disuse and which is reversed by active use, or the generalized type secondary to Cushing's syndrome or thyrotoxicosis.

There is a large group of patients, usually elderly, whose bones are unusually prone to fracturing and appear on X-ray to be less dense than those of a normal person. Bone biopsy, however, shows that the architecture and mineralization is normal. Therefore we are forced to the conclusion that such a patient has a normally formed skeleton but that there is just less of it than in a normal subject. To this condition the name osteoporosis is given.

Clinical features

These patients usually present because of a pathological fracture or because of back pain. The fracture will give the characteristic findings and usually the back pain is associated with a greater than normal degree of kyphosis. The patient may also mention that he or she is shorter than he or she used to be—often to the extent of 5–7 cm.

Radiography

A generalized lack of bone density is seen. The lumbar vertebral bodies are more biconcave than normal so that the intervertebral disc space appears more spherical (Fig. 11.5). This shape of vertebral body is seen in fishes and consequently they are referred to as 'fish vertebrae'.

In patients complaining of back pain, collapsed or wedged vertebral bodies are commonly seen. This configuration is due to porotic crush fractures of the vertebral bodies.

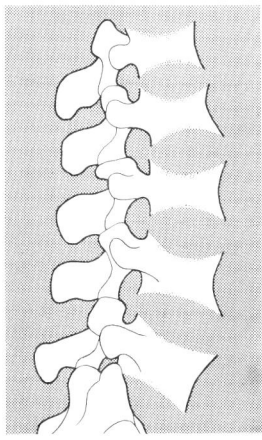

FIG. 11.5. The radiographic appearance of the lumbar vertebrae in osteoporosis.

Special investigations
Serum calcium, phosphorus, and alkaline phosphatase are usually normal. The normal alkaline phosphatase is used in some Metabolic Units to distinguish this condition from osteomalacia. Bone biopsy shows normal bone structure. Critical intake and output balance studies may show that, over a prolonged period, a negative calcium balance exists.

Treatment
The fractures are treated in the same way as similar fractures in normal bones. Diet is supplemented where necessary and it is our practice to try to reverse the negative calcium balance by giving large doses of calcium supplement (3 g per day) and an anabolic steroid. This treatment has to be continued for many months, and a careful check should be kept on renal function, particularly if vitamin D is given in addition. In occasional cases renal failure may be precipitated.

In undergraduate teaching it has always been customary to discuss osteomalacia and osteoporosis together but they have been separated here because their aetiology is different and students tend to become confused if they are discussed together.

Fibrous dysplasia of bone
This condition is included under the heading of 'unknown aetiology' because it is not truly a tumour and is not congenital.

Fibrous dysplasia may affect one bone (monostotic) or many bones (polyostotic). It is believed that the condition results from disorganization of the tissue differentiation and modelling of the diaphyses. The shafts are usually thickened and may be painful. Radiographs show irregular ossification and cystic areas. Deformity of the bone may be severe. Biopsy shows predominantly fibrous tissue and disorganization of the lamellar structure.

The prognosis for life is not affected but pathological fractures may occur. They have a normal healing potential.

There is no specific treatment for this condition.

RECOMMENDATIONS FOR FURTHER READING

COLLINS, D. H. (1966) *Pathology of Bone*, Butterworth, London.
FAIRBANK, T. (1951) *An Atlas of General Affections of the Skeleton*, Williams & Wilkins, Baltimore and E. & S. Livingstone, Edinburgh.
KING, J. D. and BOBECHKO, W. P. (1971) Osteogenesis Imperfecta—an orthopaedic description and surgical review. *J. Bone Jt Surg.* **53B**, 72–89.
PRICE, C. H. G. and GOLDIE, W. (1969) Paget's sarcoma of bone. *J. Bone Jt Surg.* **51B**, 205–24.
RANG, M. (1966) Original description of Paget's disease. In *Anthology of Orthopaedics*, pp. 19–24, E. & S. Livingstone, Edinburgh.
RANG, M. (1966) Ollier's Disease, original description. In *Anthology of Orthopaedics*, p. 25, E. & S. Livingstone, Edinburgh.
RANG, M. (1969) *The Growth Plate and its Disorders*, E. & S. Livingstone, Edinburgh.

12 Conditions of tendons and tendon sheaths

TENOSYNOVITIS

Definition
Tenosynovitis is an inflammation of the synovial sheath of a tendon. Three main types are encountered in orthopaedics:
(1) acute suppurative tenosynovitis;
(2) subacute tenosynovitis, usually affecting multiple tendons;
(3) chronic or stenosing type, sometimes referred to as 'tenosynovitis stenosans'.

Acute suppurative tenosynovitis
This is most commonly seen in the sheaths of the tendons of the long finger flexors.

Cause
Infection spreading from septic wounds of the fingers.

Symptoms
Pain spreading up the finger towards the wrist.

Signs
There may be excruciating pain on attempted extension of the finger and point tenderness over the affected tendon sheath, best elicited by pressing over the sheath with the point of a pencil or other semi-blunt object. The thenar or mid-palmar space may be inflamed and there is often swelling of the dorsum of the hand due to lymphatic spread from the palm. The regional lymph nodes may be involved.

Special investigations
Systemic signs of infection—raised erythrocyte sedimentation rate and white cell count—are usually present.

Treatment
Elevation of the hand and the administration of antibiotics are usually successful in mild and early cases. In established infections and those in which no response to antiobiotics has been obtained in 24 hours, surgical drainage of the tendon sheath is indicated.
    Finger movements should be encouraged as soon as possible in cases treated either conservatively or operatively.

Results
In early cases complete resolution usually occurs. If suppuration has occurred some stiffness of the joints moved by the tendon is almost inevitable. Severe cases may finally require amputation of the affected fingers.

Subacute tenosynovitis
This group contains several types of tenosynovitis.

Cause
This is usually obscure. Many of the patients are found in later years to be suffering from rheumatoid disease.

Symptoms
Pain, usually mild, is felt over the affected tendons on excessive use and some stiffness of the joints controlled by these tendons is noted, especially in the early mornings.

Signs
There is swelling over the tendons which is not usually tender. Characteristically, crepitus can be felt on palpating the tendon sheaths. Common sites affected are the tendons of the extensors of the wrists and fingers, the tendo-Achilles, and the peroneal tendons.

Special investigations
These are usually negative, but occasionally there are signs of rheumatic disease—a raised erythrocyte sedimentation rate and a positive rheumatoid agglutination test.

Treatment
The mainstay of treatment for this condition is rest, which can be achieved by means of splintage, e.g. a 'cock-up' splint for the wrist. If the condition continues in spite of rest, then heat and local injections of hydrocortisone acetate may be beneficial.

Results
The condition responds well to rest. Persistence in spite of treatment increases the likelihood of a rheumatoid aetiology and the condition should be treated accordingly.

Chronic tenosynovitis (tenosynovitis stenosans)
In this condition the sheath of the tendon becomes thickened and constricts the enclosed tendon.

Cause
Most cases are idiopathic, but some cases later develop other signs of rheumatoid disease. Mild cases are occasionally due to swelling following excessive unusual use of a particular tendon.

Pathology
At operation fibrous thickening of the sheath is usually found.

Symptoms
These are as follows:
1. Pain over the affected tendon sheath.
2. Evidence of interference with tendon action. In cases in which the finger flexor tendons are involved, for instance, there is classically a resistance to extension. Extra effort overcomes the obstruction—often with a sudden click—hence the expression 'trigger finger'.

Signs
Thickening of the tendon sheath is often palpable and tender, e.g. the sheath of extensor pollicis brevis in de Quervain's syndrome. The 'triggering' of the tendon may be visible, but is often more obvious when the patient actively uses the tendon than when it is moved passively. The condition occasionally affects the sheath of flexor pollicis longus in babies but is more common in middle age.

Treatment
Mild cases respond to injection of hydrocortisone acetate into the affected sheath. Severe cases and recurrent cases should be treated by excision of the thickened sheath.

Rupture of tendons
Spontaneous rupture of tendons occurs particularly in middle-aged and elderly patients. The tendon involved usually shows some sign of previous degeneration.

Cause
In the degenerative type some mild trauma, e.g. stepping down an extra step unexpectedly, usually causes the tendon to rupture.

Rheumatoid disease causes spontaneous rupture, particularly of the finger extensor tendons.

Signs
The patient cannot carry out the relevant movement of the joint and, if the examination is done soon after the rupture has occurred, the gap in the tendon may be palpable. Common tendons affected are the biceps brachii (the tendon of the long head ruptures at the level of the shoulder joint), the quadriceps expansions (just above the patella), the supraspinatus tendon and the tendo-Achilles.

Treatment
Operative repair should be carried out—the results are usually satisfactory.
Division of tendons in the hand is discussed in Chapter 24.

TUMOURS OF TENDON SHEATHS

Ganglia
The commonest tumour encountered in orthopaedic practice, this tumour arises from the synovium of joints and tendon sheaths.

Pathology
A ganglion consists of a cyst lined by a single layer of cells containing a glairy

colourless fluid. It is probably a myxomatous degeneration of synovial cells.

Symptoms
Some aching is common at the site of the swelling. Rarely, a ganglion may press on a peripheral nerve, e.g. the ulnar nerve at the wrist, giving rise to paraesthesia and paresis in the area of distribution of the nerve.

Signs
The common sites for these rubbery, lobulated, and translucent swellings are the dorsal surfaces of the wrists, hands, and feet. Occasionally one may occur near the joint line of the knee and be confused with a cyst of the meniscus.

Treatment
The time-honoured practice of bursting a ganglion by 'smiting it with the family Bible' still has its supporters, but most surgeons advise operative removal of these tumours. Recurrences are relatively common (approximately 5–10 per cent).

Giant cell tumours of tendon sheath
These tumours occur in the fingers of young adults and have recently become the object of further study because of their histological similarity to villonodular synovitis.

Symptoms
They are usually painless.

Signs
The tumour affects either the flexor or the extensor aspect of the finger. It is rubbery in consistency, lobulated, and may encircle the finger.

Radiographs
These may show some erosion of the underlying bone.

Treatment
Excision results in cure.

Benign synoviomas
These are benign tumours arising from the synovial lining of a joint or a tendon sheath.

Signs
A non-tender swelling is noticed near a joint.

Differential diagnosis
The swelling is to be distinguished from a ganglion, a bursa containing fluid, or cystic degeneration of a meniscus.

Histology
Synovial cells are seen surrounded by a collagenous matrix. Clefts lined by a single layer of synovial cells are common.

Treatment
These tumours are treated by excision. They may recur locally on occasion.

Malignant synovioma

The clinical presentation of these tumours is the same as the benign type except that occasional examples occur in unexpected places, e.g. in the ligamentum nuchae.

Histology
Characteristically two types of cells are seen:
1. The synovial cell, giving the tumour the histological appearance of a carcinoma.
2. The fibrous matrix cell, giving the appearance of a fibrosarcoma. Extension into surrounding tissue is common.

Pathology
Spread of these tumours is via the blood-stream. The patient eventually succumbs to pulmonary metastases.

Treatment
As these tumours are not radiosensitive the only hope of a cure is by excision.

Prognosis
Few patients survive 5 years.

RECOMMENDATIONS FOR FURTHER READING

CADE, S. (1962–3) Synovial sarcoma, *Jl R. Coll. Surg. Edinb.* **8**, 1–51.
RANG, M. (1966) Original description of de Quervain's stenosing Tenovaginitis. In *Anthology of Orthopaedics*, pp. 115–17, E. & S. Livingstone, Edinburgh.

13 Bone and soft-tissue tumours

The tumours encountered by the orthopaedic surgeon occur in the bones of the skeleton and in the soft tissues, mainly in the limbs. They will be considered separately.

BONE TUMOURS

There is no easy introduction to the subject of bone tumours. This is mainly due to the fact that we cannot classify these tumours satisfactorily.

Classification of tumours into groups according to cells of origin is often impossible because several cell types may occur in the same tumour, and classification into benign and malignant categories is misleading, because first the degree of malignancy is often difficult to judge microscopically, and secondly some tumours previously thought to be benign, e.g. the 'benign giant cell tumour', have later been found to metastasize.

For these reasons we shall not start out with a classification but shall be content to describe the tumours as they occur, noting any relationship a particular tumour may have with other tumours or with other conditions as we go along.

Osteomas

These are tumours arising from the osteocyte series, and are usually benign. They may consist of dense cortical bone (ivory osteomas) or normally trabeculated bone (cancellous osteomas). The latter are seen both in the long bones, e.g. femur and metacarpals, and the flat bones, e.g. pelvis and scapula.

Ivory osteomas
These occur mainly on the flat bones of the skull—they are hard flat tumours, usually on the vault, and rarely require treatment. Excision is curative.

Cancellous osteomas (exostoses, osteochondromas)
These tumours usually present in adolescents and consist of slender outgrowths of bone usually arising in the metaphyseal region and hence being found near joints.

Pathology. The tumour consists of a narrow-based, smooth, finger-like outgrowth from the metaphysis, usually extending obliquely towards the centre of the diaphysis. A cap of cartilage thought to be an ectopic area of metaphysis is found at the apex during the growth phase of the bone.

In some children, multiple tumours affecting several bones are found. The

condition is then referred to as multiple exostoses or diaphyseal aclasia—a misnomer because the lesions are really metaphyseal in position.
Cancellous tumours are also found to arise from the flat bones of the pelvis and scapulae—here the tumour is squat and flatter than in the long-bone type, and usually referred to as an osteochondroma. The cartilage cap is again present and malignant change is relatively more common than in the 'long-bone' type.

Treatment. Excision is indicated if a tumour is causing symptoms, the common example being interference with tendon action by tumours near a joint, e.g. the knee. Biopsy excision of any osteoma thought to have become malignant is also indicated. Subsequent treatment depends on the result of the biopsy.

Osteosarcomas

Malignant tumours arising from the osteocyte series are called osteosarcomas. They may be primary, as seen in young people, or secondary to other conditions such as Paget's disease or previously existing osteochondromas, in both of which cases an older age group is affected. We would recommend the term 'osteosarcoma' rather than 'osteogenic sarcoma' as the latter leads to ambiguity.

Primary osteosarcoma
A tumour occurring mainly in the metaphyseal region of the bones of young people and having a very poor prognosis.

Pathology. The commonest sites affected are the lower end of femur, the upper end of the tibia, and the upper end of the humerus. The patient is most commonly a young child, but the tumour may occur at any time up to the closure of the epiphyseal lines. It is rarely seen after the age of 20 years. As the tumour grows it expands the cortex of the bone and later erupts through it into the soft tissues. The skin over the tumour becomes distended and the whole tumour warm. Distention and proliferation of the subcutaneous veins is seen. The histological appearance of these tumours varies greatly from tumour to tumour and even in different parts of the same tumour. Since osteocytes, chondrocytes, and fibrocytes all develop from the same primitive mesenchymal cell it is not surprising that immature types of all these cells may be found. This sometimes leads to difficulty in deciding what name to give the tumour—in such cases the clinical features are helpful. As with most tumours, those containing the most anaplastic cells have the worse prognosis.

Symptoms. The patient, or the parents, usually seek advice because they have noticed a swelling. Although aching is felt, severe pain is rare in the early stages. There may be swelling of the neighbouring joint.

Signs. The bone is expanded, slightly tender, and may be warm. The signs are usually minimal in the early stages; general malaise or upset is rare. Later the tumour becomes larger and the child becomes apprehensive. Cachexia and debility are common in late cases.

Radiographs. Classically the findings on radiography are expansion of the bone

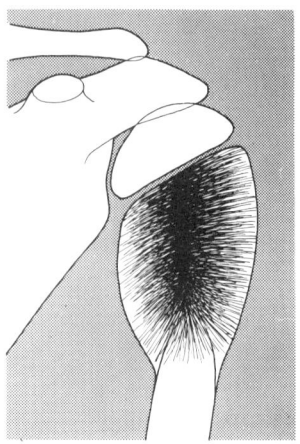

FIG. 13.1. The radiographic appearance of an osteosarcoma of the upper metaphysis of the humerus.

outline by an area of increased radiolucency, although dense areas may occur within it (Fig. 13.1). The tumour may extend into the soft tissue, showing resultant breaks in the cortical outline. The periosteum is raised by the tumour and subsequent deposition of new bone causes the formation on X-ray of triangular areas of ossification at the periphery of the tumour (Codman's triangles).

New bone is also laid down radially giving the appearance of 'sun-ray' spicules. Occasionally the tumour may present on X-ray as an area of increased density without much distortion of the bone outline. This occurs most commonly in the upper tibia.

Treatment. The majority of orthopaedic surgeons follow the line of treatment recommended by Cade. A large dose of deep X-ray therapy is given to the tumour and the patient then examined periodically. If at the end of about 6 months there is no evidence of metastases the limb is amputated. The philosophy behind this treatment is that many of these tumours have metastasized by the time the patient comes for initial treatment although these metastases may be too small to show on the chest X-ray. By waiting the period of 6 months one gives them time to become obvious. Further spread of the tumour, both local and metastatic is prevented by the deep X-ray therapy. In this way, we avoid amputation, which is very harrowing to the child, in a case of short life expectancy.

Some surgeons carry out early amputation. It is essential that a biopsy specimen is examined to establish the diagnosis before amputation is performed.

Prognosis. The early metastatic spread accounts for the bad prognosis. With any type of treatment the 5-year survival rate is well below 10 per cent.

Secondary osteosarcoma
These tumours arise commonly in Paget's disease, or, less commonly, in osteochondromas. In the former the diagnosis is usually made late in the condition because Paget's disease itself causes aching and deformity of bone.

Elevation of the serum alkaline phosphatase, which is often used in other conditions as confirmatory evidence of malignant degeneration, may well be raised in uncomplicated Paget's disease. Estimation of the urinary excretion of hydroxyprolines may be helpful.

Any increase in size or the onset of pain in an osteochondroma should suggest the diagnosis of malignant degeneration. It is more likely to occur in those tumours affecting flat bones.

Parosteal sarcomas

Pathologists have separated these tumours from osteosarcomas as they do have some distinctive features.
1. They occur in adolescents and young adults.
2. They arise from the osteoblastic layer of the periosteum and so lie alongside rather than within the bone.
3. Pain and pathological fractures are rare.
4. The tumour appears denser than the adjacent normal bone.
5. Metastases occur later than in the case of osteosarcomas. The prognosis is therefore better.

Fibroma

The benign tumour arising from the fibrocyte is a rare finding in bone, but does occur. It may cause pain in the long bones—usually in the metaphyseal region. Children and adolescents constitute the group usually affected.

Characteristically the X-rays show a rounded or bubble-shaped area of loss of bone substance surrounded by a thin line of sclerosis. The diagnosis is usually made by biopsy. Malignant change has not been reported.

The tumour is also referred to as a 'non-ossifying' fibroma or a 'cortical fibrous defect'.

Fibrosarcoma

Two main types of this malignant tumour are seen.
1. A tumour arising within the bone (*endosteal fibrosarcoma*) which grows outwards destroying bone as it goes. Cases of these tumours have been reported in Paget's disease. Spread is via the blood-stream to the lungs and to the local lymph nodes. Some are radiosensitive, others are treated by amputation. The overall 5-year survival rate is 25 per cent.
2. A tumour arising from the fibrous layer of the periosteum. This type is called a '*periosteal fibrosarcoma*' and tends to grow into the soft tissue and hence not invade the underlying bone. It is usually not sensitive to X-ray therapy but, since distant metastases are relatively rare, treatment by wide local excision or amputation is usually successful. Local recurrence may occur.

It is sometimes difficult to distinguish between a fibrous tumour of bone and monostotic fibrous dysplasia (see p. 66).

Chondromas

Chondromas are tumours of cartilage, usually found within the outline of a bone, particularly in the metaphyseal region. They occur in the long bones and also commonly in the bones of the fingers.

Symptoms and signs. They are usually painless and are often not noticed by the

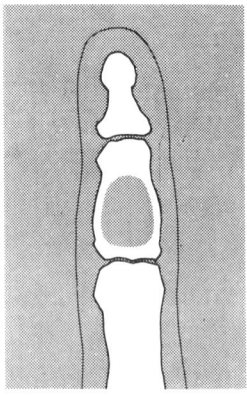

FIG. 13.2. Radiographic appearance of a chondroma of the middle phalanx of a finger.

patient unless they are the site of a pathological fracture. The swellings are clinically obvious, attached to bone, and are not tender. In the hands they may be multiple and cause unsightly swellings. If multiple tumours confined to one side of the body are present the condition is referred to as multiple enchondromarosis or Ollier's disease (dyschondroplasia).

Radiographs. These show translucent islands in the affected bones (Fig. 13.2). Later in the disease these islands show spotty areas of calcification. The pelvis may show radiating streaky areas. Growth of bone is interfered with and deformities are common.

Treatment. Excision or curettage and bone grafting usually results in a cure.

Prognosis. Malignant degeneration does occur—often after many years, and mainly in the long bones. Malignant degeneration of chondromas in the hand is excessively rare. It should be considered in any chondroma which either increases rapidly in size or becomes painful.

Chondrosarcoma

Definition. A malignant tumour mainly affecting individuals aged 20–50 years. The details of this tumour are probably most easily remembered if it is compared and contrasted with osteosarcoma.

Pathology. The tumour usually arises in long bones, the pelvis, or the scapula. Although chondromas are common in the small bones of the fingers, malignant degeneration in this site is rare. The tumour is less aggressive than the osteosarcoma and may arise in a previous chondroma. Histologically there may be some difficulty in actually deciding the actual tissue type but the difficulty is less marked than in the case of the osteosarcoma. Immature cartilage cells, often with areas of cartilage matrix, are often seen.

Symptoms. The patient usually complains of mild but gradually increasing pain felt deep in the limb. There may have been a swelling present at the site—often for many years. Pathological fractures occasionally occur.

Signs. The swelling is usually palpable and slightly tender and there may be soft tissue swelling over it.

Radiographs. Classically the tumour presents an area of loss of bone density and, within it, speckles of calcification. The cortex may be destroyed in some areas but 'sun-ray spicules' and Codman's triangle are not commonly seen. In some patients there is very little to be seen on radiography other than a small area of diminished bone density with preservation of most of the trabecular pattern.

Treatment. These tumours are rarely radiosensitive and if there is no sign of spread to distant sites, amputation should be undertaken if at all possible.

Prognosis. Compared again to osteosarcoma the prognosis of chondrosarcoma is relatively good: the 5-year survival rate is over 50 per cent.

Ewing's tumour

This is a highly malignant tumour affecting children between the ages of 5 years and 15 years.

Origin. This has not yet been completely clarified, hence the eponymous name. Most authorities accept that it arises from the endothelium of the marrow spaces, but there is a considerable body of opinion which holds that this tumour may be a metastasis from a neuroblastoma.

Occurrence. The condition is commonest between the ages of 5 years and 15 years and occurs in both sexes equally. The femur, tibia, and humerus are most commonly affected, in that order of frequency, but the tumour may also be seen in flat bones (e.g. pelvis or ribs).

Symptoms. Pain felt in the centre of the shaft of a long bone.

Signs. A tender swelling in the midshaft of the bone. Fever and leucocytosis are common.

Radiographs. These show a characteristic area of increased radiolucency (bone destruction) with layers of periosteal new bone laid down around it—the 'onion-peel appearance'.

Appearance. The macroscopic appearance is of a soft, highly vascular tumour. When examined micropscopically, a very cellular tumour consisting of round cells is seen.

Differential diagnosis. Pyogenic osteomyelitis and syphilis must be excluded.

Treatment. Amputation after biopsy is recommended. Some tumours respond to radiotherapy for a limited period.

Prognosis. There is a very poor prognosis—there are virtually no 5-year survivors.

Giant cell tumours of bone

The origin of this tumour has been the subject of controversy for years. It has been believed in the past that the tumour arose from the osteoclast—hence the old name 'osteoclastoma'. It was also believed to be benign and for this reason was referred to by some as the 'benign giant cell tumour'. The present view is first that there is no good evidence to support the theory that the giant cells—which are undoubtedly present—are derived from osteoclasts, and secondly that the behaviour of some of these tumours is anything but benign. So we are left with a descriptive name 'giant cell tumour of bone' and the knowledge that these tumours may be either benign or malignant.

Pathology. The tumours usually occur between the ages of 20 years and 40 years. Sex incidence is equal. Giant cell tumours usually affect the ends of long bones, showing a predilection for the lower end of the femur and radius and the upper end of the tibia and humerus. The overlying cortex is thinned and, in the days before early diagnosis, could often be cracked like an egg-shell by the examiner. On section the tumour is found to be vacuolated in structure and to contain red vascular tumour tissue and areas of fat.

Histological examination reveals two main characteristics, the multi-nucleate cells and a stroma containing spindle-shaped and oval cells.

It is now believed that the malignant potential of these tumours lies in the stromal cells and the tumours are therefore graded according to the degree of anaplasia of the stromal cells.

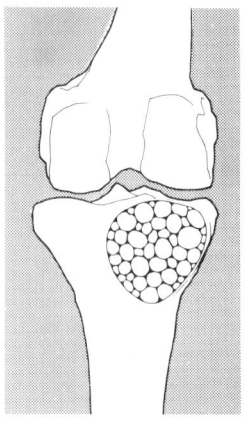

FIG. 13.3. The radiographic appearance of a giant cell tumour of the upper tibia.

Symptoms. Aching, pain, and restriction of movement of the neighbouring joint are common.

Signs. The expanded end of the bone may be visible and palpable. It is usually warm. Pathological fracture may occur through the tumour.

Radiographs. Radiographs show a characteristic 'soap-bubble' or 'foamy' appearance of the tumour—usually eccentrically placed in the early stages but later filling the whole thickness of the bone and expanding and thinning the cortex (Fig. 13.3). The tumour extends right up to the subchondral bone of the end of the bone affected.

Treatment. If practical, excision of the affected area of bone, e.g. the upper end of the fibula, should be done. If this is not feasible the choice lies between deep X-ray therapy (many tumours are radiosensitive) and curetting the lesion and packing the resulting space with bone chips. Occasionally excision of the tumour and arthrodesis of the neighbouring joint are carried out.

Prognosis. Local recurrence is common except after excision. Blood-spread metastatic lesions do occur in up to about 25 per cent of cases in reported series.

Myeloma
Solitary myeloma and multiple myelomatosis
The alternative name of these tumours is 'plasmacytoma', and this helps in remembering the cell type found on histology. Occasionally a patient is found to have a single tumour and is cured by its excision. More often, however, multiple tumours are found and the condition is referred to as multiple myelomatosis.

Pathology. The condition affects the 40–60 year-old group and men are affected twice as commonly as women. The 'marrow bones' (the long bones of the limbs, skull, sternum, and pelvis and spine) are usually involved.

Histology reveals highly cellular types, the cells being plasmacytes which are oval cells with nuclei showing the characteristic 'cart-wheel' arrangement of chromatin.

Symptoms. The commonest presenting symptom is backache but pain in other bones is also encountered.

Signs. Tenderness in affected bones may be present and pathological fractures are seen.

Special investigations. These are as follows:
1. *Urine.* 50–60 per cent of patients show the characteristic Bence–Jones proteose in the urine. This substance precipitates out on heating the urine to 60 °C and redissolves if heating is continued.
2. *Plasma proteins.* The plasma proteins show an increase in the globulin fraction which may be large enough to reverse the albumin–globulin ratio. Electrophoresis show a dense band in the gammaglobulin section to which the name 'M-band' has been applied.
3. *Sternal marrow biopsy.* The findings here are usually conclusive—the marrow shows the presence of myeloma cells. However, the marrow may be normal in cases of solitary myeloma.

Radiographs. Classically these show circular 'punched-out' areas of radiolucency in bone, particularly in the skull and pelvis. The areas are of varying sizes.

Treatment. Radiotherapy gives temporary relief but no curative treatment has yet been found with the exception of excision of the solitary lesion.

Leukaemia

The blood-forming tissues of the bone marrow may undergo malignant change resulting in the conditions of myeloid and lymphatic leukaemia. These conditions are better studied in haematology textbooks.

The orthopaedic surgeon is, however, occasionally confronted by a patient with an X-ray showing the findings of leukaemia:
(1) the patient is usually a child;
(2) there is generalized reduction of bone density;
(3) flame-shaped areas of loss of bone substance are seen at the metaphyses.

Osteoid osteoma

This condition occurs in patients between 10 years and 30 years of age. It is not certain whether or not it is a tumour in the accepted sense of the word.

Symptoms. The patient complains of pain and can usually localize it exactly. The femur and tibia are the commonest sites but the condition can occur in any bone except the skull. Classically the pain is worse at night and is relieved by aspirin.

Signs. If the affected bone is superficial, a thickening may be felt. The swelling may be warm and tender. If the spine is affected the movement may be restricted but tenderness will probably not be elicited.

Radiographs. Early in the condition radiography may show increase in the cortical thickness of a bone. Later, the area of 'sclerotic' bone becomes larger and an area of increased radiolucency becomes evident in its centre. This phenomenon is referred to as a 'nidus'. Tomography may be necessary to demonstrate a nidus.

Pathology. Some authorities believe that osteoid osteomas are caused by chronic infection, but all attempts to demonstrate an infecting organism or any systemic signs of infection have been unsuccessful.

Treatment. Excision of the nidus cures the condition. The nidus may be difficult to find at operation and radiography may be required during the procedure.

Prognosis. Recurrence and metastases have not been reported after excision of the nidus.

Aneurysmal bone cyst

This is actually a vascular tumour occuring in bone. It affects children and appears in the metaphysis as a cystic lesion containing blood lying in large spaces lined with endothelium.

Radiographs reveal the cyst with, on occasion, periosteal new bone laid down over it. The cyst may have trabeculae crossing it. Excision and packing with bone chips is the treatment of choice.

Metastases in bone

It should be emphasized that all the above tumours, with the possible exception of myelomatosis and leukaemia, are primarily of bone cells.

Secondary deposits from tumours in other parts of the body are, in fact, much more common than primary bone tumours and the commoner sites of primary tumours spreading to the skeleton via the blood-stream are breast, lung, kidney, thyroid, and prostate. Most secondary deposits are osteolytic (bone-destroying) but metastases from carcinoma of the prostate and, very rarely, those from carcinoma of the breast may be osteosclerotic. Skeletal deposits from prostatic carcinoma are, in the vast majority of cases accompanied by a rise in the serum 'prostatic' acid phosphatase level.

SOFT-TISSUE TUMOURS

Although comparatively rare, soft-tissue tumours do occur in orthopaedic practice from time to time. The main reason for this is that most of them present as swelling situated in the limbs and differentiation from cysts and ganglia is difficult.

Ganglia and synoviomata have been dealt with in Chapter 12 (p. 67) and neuromata in Chapter 5 (p. 25). This section deals with vascular tumours and tumours of the muscle and fibrous tissue.

Vascular tumours

Glomus tumours
These present usually in middle-aged patients as small swellings, particularly on the hand. The outstanding characteristic is their extreme tenderness to touch or pressure. Excision is curative.

Arterio-venous aneurysms
The development of peripheral vascular surgery has relieved the orthopaedic surgeon from having to deal with the majority of these tumours. He does, however, encounter them as diagnostic problems: those situated more proximally in the limb may give rise to limb-length discrepancies and those occurring more distally may cause ischaemia of fingers and toes. The detailed investigation (arteriograms) and treatment is now done in vascular surgery units.

Tumours of muscle

Smooth muscle tumours
The benign variety (leiomyoma) is encountered as a swelling in the limb which on exploration may be found to be intimately connected to a blood-vessel. The diagnosis may be suspected at operation but can be conclusively proved only by histological examination.

The malignant variety (leiomyosarcoma) tends to recur locally after excision rather than to metastasize. Deep X-ray therapy is usually given after excision.

Striated muscle tumours
Both the benign type (rhabdomyoma) and the malignant type (rhabdomyosarcoma) are very rare and, in the latter, local recurrence is more likely than distant spread. For the malignant type prophylactic deep X-ray therapy is given after excision.

Experience with these tumours suggests that recurrence is associated with the reversion to a more primitive type of cell. This is also seen in recurrence of fibrosarcomas (see below). Consequently any unit dealing with a significant number of these tumours tends to adopt the terminology of 'round-cell sarcoma' for the recurrences containing more primitive cell types.

The difficult decision for the surgeon is the point at which amputation of the limb should be advised. No hard and fast rule can be made on this point and even when they are advised to have a limb amputated, most patients have great difficulty with accepting such advice.

Tumours of fibrous tissue

Fibroma
True benign tumours arising from fibrous tissue are excessively rare—most of the tumours previously thought to be pure fibromas were probably neurofibromas.

Fibrosarcoma
The malignant tumour of fibrous tissue is however occasionally encountered although the histologist may have difficulty in deciding whether the tumour under consideration is in fact a fibrosarcoma or represents a reversion to a more primitive cell type.

Treatment is by wide excision followed by a course of deep X-ray therapy. Recurrence is, unfortunately, not rare and amputation may be indicated.

RECOMMENDATIONS FOR FURTHER READING

CADE, S. (1962–3) Synovial sarcoma, *J. R. Coll. Surg. Edinb.* **8**, 1–51.
EYRE-BROOK, A. L. and PRICE, C. H. G. (1969) Fibrosarcoma of bone, *J. Bone Jt Surg.* **51B**, 20–37.
MCGRATH, P. J. (1972) Giant cell tumour of bone, *J. Bone Jt Surg.* **54B**, 216–29.
SWEETNAM, R. (1963) Osteosarcoma, *Ann. R. Coll. Surg.* **44**, 38–58.

General reference
LICHTENSTEIN, L. (1972) *Bone Tumours*, C. V. Mosby, Saint Louis.

14 Other conditions of joints

In this chapter we shall cover those conditions of joints not discussed in other chapters:
 (1) gout;
 (2) osteochondritis dissecans;
 (3) arthrogryphosis multiplex congenita;
 (4) loose bodies in joints;
 (5) villonodular synovitis;
 (6) synovial chondromatosis;
 (7) Charcot's disease.

Gout

There are a number of people whose metabolism of purine is deficient and whose serum contains an excess of uric acid. If this situation is found in combination with painful joints the condition is called gout. The pain in the joints is caused by the deposition of urate crystals and the reaction of the joint may be severe, sometimes being clinically indistinguishable from acute septic arthritis. More often, however, the joints become subacutely inflamed and present a diagnostic problem.

Clinical features
The joint characteristically affected is the metatarso-phalangeal joint of the big toe. It becomes acutely tender, painful, warm, red, and swollen. More commonly, however, the disease affects several joints, e.g. the small joints of the hands or the feet. Occasionally one large joint, perhaps the knee or ankle, is affected. In the majority of cases the inflammation of the joint is more subacute in character and differentiation from rheumatoid disease may be difficult, The presence of urate depositions in other parts of the body as 'tophi' is not, in fact, common but if they are found, e.g. on the ears, the diagnosis is made easier.
 In rare cases, gross swelling of the peri-articular tissues due to uric-acid crystal deposition is seen.

Special investigations
The serum uric acid is usually raised above the normal level of 6 mg per 100 ml. The normal value varies a little from laboratory to laboratory but values of 7 mg per 100 ml and over are definitely significant. It is important to stress that hyperuricaemia may occur in patients who do not have any joint involvement, but in those with joint involvement, symptomatic relief usually occurs when the serum uric acid is lowered. Microscopic examination of the fluid aspirated from an affected joint may reveal the characteristic needle-shaped crystals of uric acid.

Radiographs
These may show a generalized osteoporosis of the area involved and, later in the condition, small bone cysts appear in the bones near the involved joints.

Treatment
The treatment of gout is aimed at correcting the results of the metabolic deficiency by reducing the level of circulating uric acid. This may be achieved by increasing its excretion using probenacid, salicylates, or phenylbutazone, or reducing its production by the administration of allopurinol.

In acute attacks the classical treatment by the administration of colchicine is still used on occasion but there is a high probability that the patient will suffer nausea and may vomit when it is given. As there is a danger of renal damage in prolonged hyperuricaemia, some physicians recommend permanent use of drugs to keep the uric-acid level within normal limits.

Repeated or prolonged joint affection may lead to articular cartilage destruction and subsequent osteoarthrosis.

Osteochondritis dissecans

This condition is seen predominantly in adolescents and young adults. It is of unknown aetiology and various theories as to its causation have been advanced. Essentially it consists of the necrosis of an area of bone adjacent to a joint surface, with accompanying death of the deeper layers of the overlying articular cartilage. This may or may not lead to separation of this segment of bone and cartilage. The name was introduced in the late 1800s because it was felt that an area of inflammation developed between the living and the dead bone and that this inflammation 'dissected' out the dead area and caused it to separate.

Clinical features
The joints most commonly affected are the knee, the elbow, and the ankle. There are also occasional reports of the hip joint being involved. In the early stages of the disease the patient complains of pain in the affected joint but physical examination and radiography do not reveal any abnormalities. As the condition progresses, however, the dead area of bone becomes visible on radiographs and if the segment separates the bony part of the loose 'fragment' will be visible on the films. The parts of the femur most often affected when the condition occurs in the knee are the lateral aspect of the medial femoral condyle or its weight-bearing surface (Fig. 14.1). In the elbow the capitellar surface, and in the ankle the dome of the talus are the common sites for the lesion to be found.

Once the segment has separated, the patient may suffer attacks of locking, swelling, and, in the case of the knee, 'giving way' on weight bearing. This triad of symptoms is also seen in meniscus lesions and it is for this reason that no knee is ever explored for a meniscus lesion without first being X-rayed to exclude the presence of a loose segment —usually referred to as a 'loose body'.

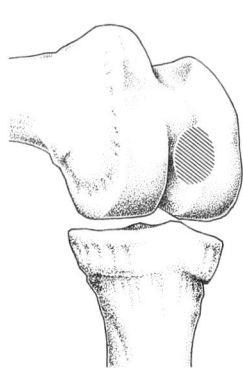

FIG. 14.1. Osteochondritis dissecans showing the common site for the ulcer on the medial femoral condyle.

Examination may reveal the loose body as a palpable movable lump and the patient may mention that he has been able to palpate it on occasion.

Treatment
If one can be sure that the segment has not separated, conservative treatment is given. This consists of rest and, if the area is in the weight-bearing part of the joint, the patient is advised not to take weight on the limb. Crutches or a weight-relieving caliper are used.

If it is felt that the segment is in danger of separating or the patient is not responding to weight relief, the area is exposed at operation and the dead bone drilled to encourage a new blood-supply. The dead area may be difficult to locate because the superficial layers of the articular cartilage over it may be of normal appearance. (The superficial layers receive their nutrition from the synovial fluid.) Pressure with a blunt probe, however, usually locates the softened area.

If the segment has separated it is removed and the crater drilled to encourage 'filling in' with fibro-cartilage. The operation is followed by a period of non-weight-bearing walking.

Results
If the necrosed area is not on a weight-bearing surface a satisfactory result is obtained. If it is, there is a possibility that degenerative arthrosis may follow. Healing of the crater does occur in many cases in which it has been drilled.

Arthrogryposis multiplex congenita

This condition is included under affections of joints because the joint deformities are the most obvious abnormalities. It is, however, in essence a defect in the development of mesenchyme resulting in a failure in the differentiation of muscles, ligaments, and tendons. Bone growth is also defective, resulting in the affected limb or limbs being shorter than normal (Fig. 14.2).

Clinical features
Deformity may be apparent at birth or soon after. Any or all of the limb joints may be affected although in some cases only the lower limbs are affected. A clue to the diagnosis may be the complete lack of creases in the skin overlying the

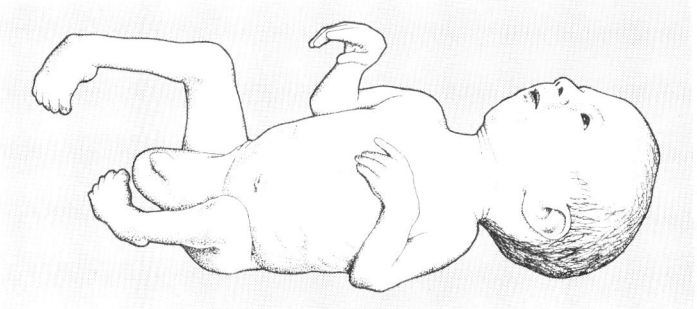

FIG. 14.2. Arthrogryposis multiplex congenita.

joints. Flexion contractures of the joints are common. Flexion and ulnar deviation of the wrist, adduction contractures of the hips, and equinovarus deformity of the ankle are also seen. The differentiation from a congenital talipes equinovarus may be difficult but the size of the heel may be a help: in CTEV the heel is usually hypoplastic.

Special investigations
The diagnosis may be proved by biopsy of the tissues involved: muscles, tendons, and ligaments are represented by undifferentiated fibrous tissue.

Treatment
The aim of treatment is to keep the deformities to a minimum and to encourage the child to make full use of the muscle and joint action which he has. Splintage in the normal position in the early months is combined with periodic manipulation and stretching.

Later, active physiotherapy is added and finally soft-tissue operations and osteotomy may be required to keep the joints in an optimum position.

Loose bodies in joints
The smooth movement of a joint may be upset by the presence of a piece of bone or cartilage lying free in the joint. This has probably separated from one of the joint surfaces, and its presence is not suspected until the joint suddenly locks (fails to extend but continues to flex), or the range of flexion is reduced. If there is a sudden interference with joint movement, reaction by the joint in the form of synovial effusion is common. The joints most commonly affected are the knee and elbow but the phenomenon is also seen in the hip, ankle, and shoulder.

If the loose body contains a calcified or an ossified portion it will be visible on radiography. Occasionally the loose body is palpable—especially if it is in the suprapatellar pouch of the knee.

The causes of loose body formation are:
(1) osteochondritis dissecans;
(2) osteoarthrosis (the separation of osteophytes);
(3) fractures;
(4) synovial chondromatosis or osteochondromatosis;
(5) Charcot's disease.

It is important to distinguish between 'loose bodies' which arises from structures normally present in the joint and 'foreign bodies' which are put into the joint from outside, e.g. pieces of glass or shrapnel fragments.

Villonodular synovitis
This is a relatively rare condition of unknown aetiology affecting most commonly the knee and elbow joint. The synovial membrane becomes hyperplastic and thrown into villi or folds. The exuberant folds may be traumatized and bleed. This causes staining of the synovium by blood pigments and a characteristic appearance at operation often referred to as pigmented villonodular synovitis. The condition is not usually painful. Involvement of the subchondral bone with cyst formation has been reported.

Aetiology
Opinion is divided amongst pathologists specializing in this subject as to whether this condition is a type of benign tumour or a low-grade inflammatory response.

Treatment
Synovectomy usually cures the condition.

Synovial chondromatosis

This condition is considered to be an example of metaplasia: the synovial cells undergo a change to chondrocytes and produce cartilaginous loose bodies within a joint. The condition starts with the formation of multiple, small, heaped-up areas on the synovial surface, the tips of which become cartilaginous and subsequently separate to lie free in the joint. Occasionally they become ossified, in which case the condition is called osteochondromatosis.

The number of loose bodies is variable but may run into many hundreds. The joints commonly affected are the knee and the shoulder.

Treatment
Removal of the loose bodies is usually combined with synovectomy to prevent recurrence.

Charcot's disease

Charcot was a French surgeon in the 1800s who described the changes in joints of patients suffering from syphilis. The changes are due to the fact that the nerve supply to the joint is deficient and his name is applied to any joint which degenerates because of neurological deficiency. The other name applied to these joints is 'neuropathic joints'.

Characteristically the joint is deformed and swollen, exhibits a very wide range of movement, and is painless. The knee is the commonest joint affected. Radiography shows a grossly disorganized joint with hypertrophy of the articular surfaces and often the presence of multiple loose bodies.

Syringomyelia may also cause the development of neuropathic joint, characteristically the elbow.

Treatment
Supporting splintage is usually advised in cases of knee involvement because of the difficulty of obtaining bony union in arthrodoesis.

Elbow involvement may require stabilization in a splint but more often does not require treatment.

RECOMMENDATIONS FOR FURTHER READING

AICHROTH, P. (1971) Osteochondritis of the knee—a clinical survey, *J. Bone Jt Surg.* **53B**, 440–7.

LLOYD-ROBERTS, G. C. and LETTIN, A. W. F. (1970) Arthrogryposis multiplex congenita, *J. Bone Jt Surg.* **52B**, 594–513.

RANG, M. (1966) Original description of Charcot's disease of joints. In *Anthology of Orthopaedics*, pp. 42–7, E. & S. Livingstone, Edinburgh.

PART II
Regional conditions

15 The neck

ANATOMY OF THE SPINE

Before considering the neck in detail, we shall discuss the anatomy of the spine in general because there are several conditions which are common to all parts of the spine.

The vertebrae

A typical vertebra consists of two main parts: the body in front; and the neural arch behind (Fig. 15.1). The bodies of the vertebrae make up two-thirds of the height of the spine and form, with the intervertebral discs, a column extending from pelvis to skull. The neural arches encircle the spinal cord and together with the ligamenta flava, the interspinous, and supraspinous ligaments form a protective cylinder around it.

The neural arch consists of a pedicle and a lamina on each side, the laminae meeting in the midline posteriorly.

Several processes of bone arise from the neural arch:
1. The transverse processes from the junction of pedicles and laminae. These lie in approximately the horizontal plane.
2. The superior and inferior articular processes, which arise from approximately the same location on the neural arch as do the transverse processes, but lie in the vertical plane.
3. The spinous process, which arises in the midline at the junction of the two laminae and lies in an obliquely downward and backward plane when seen from the lateral aspect.

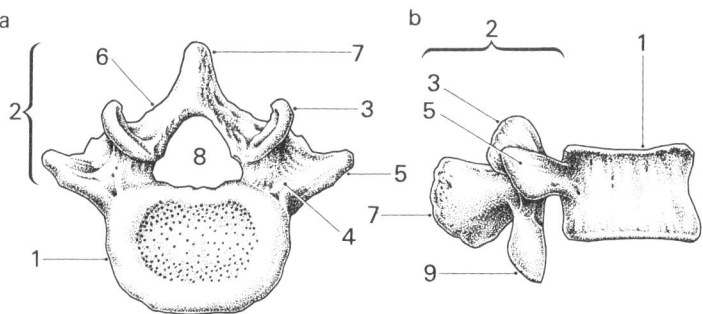

FIG. 15.1. (a) A vertebra seen from above. (b) A vertebra seen from the side: (1) body; (2) neural arch; (3) superior articular process; (4) pedicle; (5) transverse process; (6) lamina; (7) spinous process; (8) spinal canal; (9) inferior articular process.

Ossification

The vertebral body may be looked upon from the point of view of ossification as a foreshortened long bone. It ossifies from a primary centre for the main part (diaphysis), and two secondary centres for the end plates (epiphyses). These end-plate epiphyses are not complete discs but are deficient centrally, rather like flattened doughnuts, and referred to as ring epiphyses.

The neural arch ossifies from a primary centre for each side. The appearance of other secondary centres for the neural arch varies at different levels, but there is usually one for the spinous process and one for each transverse process.

The intervertebral discs

These are fibro-elastic cushions which are found between the vertebral bodies. Each one consists of a strong outer coat, or annulus fibrosis, and a softer centre, or nucleus pulposis. The discs are subject to considerable deformation strains during movements of the spine. These forces are greatest in the lower lumbar spine especially at the junction of the mobile lumbar spine and the fixed sacrum, i.e. the disc between the fifth lumbar. and the first sacral vertebrae.

The posterior joints

The joints are formed between the lower articular processes of one vertebra and the upper articular processes of the vertebra below. They are synovial joints and are therefore subject to all the conditions affecting other synovial joints, e.g. rheumatoid disease and degenerative arthrosis. They are called 'posterior joints' to distinguish them from the syndesmoses between vertebral bodies and discs which are the 'anterior joints'.

Normal curves of the spine

The normal spine is straight when viewed from the front (the antero-posterior view) but has several curves when viewed from the side (lateral view). A curve which is convex forwards is called a lordosis or lordotic curve and a curve which is convex backwards is called a kyphosis or kyphotic curve. The normal spine has the following curves:
   (1) a cervical lordosis;
   (2) a thoracic kyphosis;
   (3) a lumbar lordosis;
   (4) a sacral kyphosis.

It must be stressed that these are normal curves and are therefore different from the lateral curve or 'scoliosis' which is seen in the antero-posterior view and is always abnormal.

DEFINITIONS

There are several words which students find confusing. They all start with the prefix *spond*—meaning 'spine'.

Spondylosis

Degeneration of the spine. This term is used particularly to describe degeneration of the intervertebral discs. Degeneration of the posterior joints, which are synovial joints, is referred to as osteoarthrosis.

Spondylitis
Inflammation of the spine, which may be bacterial (e.g. tuberculous spondylitis). The term is also used in a peculiar affection of the spine which leads to stiffening (or 'ankylosis') of all the joints of the spine—'ankylosing spondylitis'.

Spondylolysis
Loss of continuity of the spine. This term is applied to a condition affecting individual vertebral bodies in which continuity of bone in the neural arch is lost and an area of fibrosis is found in the arch, usually in the area between the articular pillars—the 'pars interarticularis'.

Spondylolisthesis
In this condition one vertebral body moves forward on the body beneath it and alignment of the spine, as seen in the lateral view, is lost. It may be seen in association with a gap in the pars interarticularis or with marked osteoarthrosis and deformation of the posterior joints.

CONDITIONS AFFECTING THE NECK

Klippel–Feil syndrome
In this congenital condition the development of the vertebrae in the cervical region is deficient. There is loss of segmentation leading to a short neck with restricted movements. In severe cases the appearance of the child suggests that the head and chest are continuous with no intervening neck. The syndrome may be associated with unilateral or bilateral congenital elevation of the scapula (Sprengel's shoulder). Neurological complications are rare and there is no specific treatment for the neck condition.

Torticollis (wry-neck)
The name wry-neck is given to the condition in which the head and neck are held flexed over to one side. There may be an element of rotation present as well—the face being rotated to the opposite side to that to which the head is flexed. It is important to realize that the action of the sternomastoid is to produce flexion of the neck to its own side but rotation to the opposite side. There are three main types of torticollis.

Spasmodic torticollis
This is usually seen in young adults and is the common 'stiff-neck' syndrome. The patient usually wakes up with pain in one side of the neck and finds that the neck has become stiff and flexed to one side. Any attempted movement is painful. Examination reveals spasm of the sternomastoid and trapezius muscles.

The cause of this condition is obscure and is probably different in different patients. In some the condition follows exposure to cold, and in others it may well be due to a minor subluxation of a posterior joint, causing irritation of a spinal nerve. Most cases respond favourably to heat, especially microwave therapy, and some make an almost instantaneous recovery after gentle traction to the cervical spine. Full investigation of the cervical region should be done before advising manipulation. Symptoms may also be relieved by wearing a cervical collar.

Infantile torticollis
Restriction of neck movements and tightness of the sternomastoid muscle is often noted soon after birth. In some of these babies a swelling is palpable in the lower third of the sternomastoid just above the clavicle. This is referred to as a 'sternomastoid tumour' and is thought to be due to haemorrhage into, or infarction of, the lower fibres of the muscle, possibly during delivery. The swelling usually disappears during the first few months of life but the sternomastoid muscle may not develop and grow as well as that on the other side. This will lead to a progression of the torticollis if no treatment is given. As the child grows, secondary changes in the face and skull occur. The opposite side of the face becomes longer (particularly the mandible) and frontal bossing occurs. The final deformity may be severe.

Treatment. The aim is to preserve the length of the sternomastoid muscle. To this end, stretching of the muscle by the mother is encouraged and periodic checks are made so that any sign of contracture or secondary facial changes can be noted. If either of these develop, operative lengthening of the muscle by tenotomy is advised.

The operation is performed through an incision either at the lower end of the muscle just above the clavicle or at its upper end at the mastoid process. Exploration at the lower end often reveals that there is also tightness of other structures, e.g. the scalene muscles or the fasciae of the neck.

After operation, all cases are periodically checked and severe cases may require immobilization in the corrected position in a plaster-cast for some months.

Scoliotic torticollis
Some children suffering from torticollis may be shown on radiography to have congenital anomalies of the cervical vertebrae or to have a scoliotic curve which involves both the cervical spine and the thoracic spine.

Treatment of the scoliosis may improve the torticollis but those due to congenital anomalies in the cervical spine are usually not suitable for operative correction because of the risks involved.

Neck and upper limb pain
A very large number of patients attend orthopaedic clinics with symptoms of pain in the neck and upper limb. Characteristically the pain travels down the outer side of the upper limb, and it may be accompanied by tingling in the fingers.

A similar set of symptoms occur in the lower back and lower limb, and these will be described later. The clinical approach to these patients is identical.

The initial assessment follows very simple lines and is designed to put the patient into one of three groups:
 (1) neck pain only;
 (2) neck pain and upper limb pain (neuralgia);
 (3) neck pain and neuralgia and a neurological deficit in the upper limbs.
The reasoning behind this classification is that in groups (1) and (2) we have no evidence of root or nerve entrapment or compression. This means that the cause of the pain is in the neck or in the area of supply of the cervical segments of the cord and that the upper limb pain may be a referred pain, whereas in group (3) pain is almost certainly due to root or nerve entrapment.

Referred pain
We find two concepts of pain help us considerably in assessing these patients. There is first Hilton's dictum that if a patient has pain in an area of his body, the cause of that pain is either in that area or in the area of supply of the nerves (spinal segments) supplying the area.

Secondly, there is the whole concept of referred pain. This is really an elaboration of Hilton's dictum. A pain-producing lesion may cause pain to be felt in some part of the body other than that in which it is situated; the connection between the two parts being that they are supplied by the same spinal segment. In this way a subphrenic irritation, e.g. from blood in the peritoneum, may be felt in the shoulder, or a chronic prostatis may cause pain in the back of the thighs.

The examination of the patient therefore begins with a detailed study of the movements of the relevant area of the spine (in this case the neck). Particular note is made of any restriction of movement and whether the pain is aggravated by movement. The examiner then proceeds to a detailed neurological examination of the limbs, looking for any sign of neurological deficit.

It should be emphasized that the pain of a frozen shoulder (capsulitis) or a tennis elbow is often felt down the limb in addition to the area affected.

Cervical spondylosis
This is probably the commonest lesion to cause the syndrome of neck and upper-limb neuralgia. It is commonest after the age of 35 years and tends to affect the C5–C6 and C6–C7 discs more than the lower ones (Fig. 15.2). The pain is felt down the outer side of the upper limb and is aggravated by neck movements. Radiographs in early cases may show some narrowing of the disc spaces and in later cases show gross narrowing and the presence of osteophytes attached to the vertebral bodies. In late cases osteophytic encroachment of the intervertebral foramen may lead to pressure on the roots

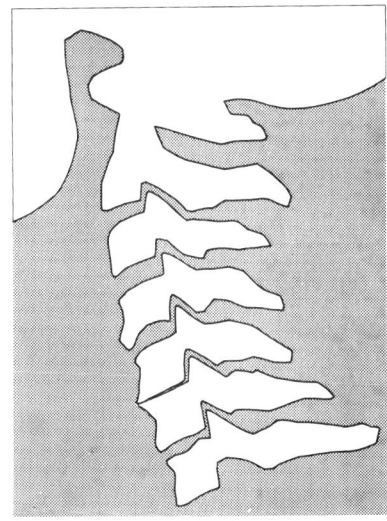

FIG. 15.2. Cervical spondylosis affecting the C5–C6 disc space.

and a neurological deficit (i.e. the patient is now in group (3) of p. 94). This is rare.

Treatment consists either in giving heat (in the form of short-wave diathermy) and asking the physiotherapists to gradually and gently mobilize the the neck, or in immobilizing the spine in a collar until the pain has passed off. This latter policy is pursued in the elderly and in severe cases.

Spinal fusion for cervical spondylosis is very seldom required and should only be used after a full course of conservative treatment has proved unsuccessful.

Acute prolapse of the intervertebral disc

As in the lumbar spine acute prolapse of an intervertebral disc is occasionally seen in the cervical spine. It is, however, much less common, and the condition usually responds to conservative measures. The pain may be very severe and debilitating and some units advise surgical removal of the disc material and bone grafting of the disc space. Because of the dangers of operating on the cervical spinal cord, this procedure is usually done from the antero-lateral aspect of the vertebral bodies.

Osteoarthrosis of the cervical spine

Degeneration of the posterior joints of the cervical spine is not uncommon in the elderly and may occur together with cervical spondylosis. Treatment is usually by collar immobilization and analgesics until the pain has settled.

The thoracic outlet syndrome

Pain radiating down the upper limb is caused occasionally by interference with the subclavian artery and the lower trunk of the brachial plexus as they pass over the first rib. The area bounded by the first ribs is known as the thoracic outlet and symptoms arising from causes in this area are referred to as the thoracic outlet syndrome.

The vessel and nerve trunk may be pressed on by tightness of the scalene muscles or by the presence of an extra rib arising from the seventh cervical vertebra and referred to as a 'cervical rib'. This may be present as a bony structure or be represented in part or whole by a fibrous band passing from the lateral mass of the seventh cervical vertebra to the first rib. The subclavian artery passes over this structure and may become acutely angulated. Movements of the shoulder girdle may cause pressure on the vessel by the clavicle.

Symptoms

The patient complains of pain down the arm and coldness and pallor of the limb. In those cases in which the nerve trunk is mainly affected the patient usually feels an aching pain down the limb, especially if she carried anything heavy, e.g. a shopping basket. Symptoms are commonest in the middle-aged.

Examination

This may reveal a neurological deficit in the limb, e.g. weakness or wasting of the intrinsic muscles of the hand or an area of sensory loss on the inner side of the upper limb. It may be possible to cause the radial pulse to disappear by putting the limb into certain positions, e.g. elevation or external rotation.

Radiographs
The plain radiograph may show the presence of the cervical rib. Angiography may demonstrate the presence of vascular narrowing in the region of the first rib. In long-standing cases there may be post-stenotic dilatation distal to the narrowing.

Treatment
Minor cases respond to conservative treatment, which consists of shrugging exercises and other exercises aimed at improving the support of the shoulder girdle. Excision of the cervical rib or release of the tight structures at the thoracic outlet should only be done in collaboration with the vascular surgeon as resection of the narrowed section of artery and replacement with a vein graft may be necessary.

INJURIES TO THE CERVICAL SPINE

Injuries to the cervical spine are common and tend to occur in falls, especially falls down stairs, and in motor traffic accidents. It is an unhappy coincidence that they are often found in combination with head injuries and are difficult to assess because the patient may be unconscious at the time of examination.

The vertebrae
There are five typical cervical vertebrae, the atlas and axis being atypical because of their shape and involvement in the movements of rotation and nodding. Inspection of a typical cervical vertebra will show that the articular facets of the posterior joints are inclined slightly upwards and forwards from the horizontal plane. This would suggest that the most common injury would be forward dislocation of one vertebra on the next below, and this is indeed the case.

The anterior surfaces of the bodies of the cervical vertebrae are attached to the strong anterior spinal ligament.

The cervical cord
Enclosed within the cervical part of the spinal canal is the caudal part of the medulla oblongata above and the cervical cord below. The segments of the cord correspond roughly with the vertebral bodies, i.e. the spinal nerves pass approximately horizontally to reach the relevant intervertebral foramina.

The phrenic nerve, the motor supply to the diaphragm, arises mainly from the fourth cervical segment and passes down the neck, lying on the anterior surface of the scalenus anterior muscle. Any injury to the spinal cord above the fourth cervical segment therefore causes immediate cessation of respiration, and death, but in an injury below the fourth cervical segment the diaphragm will continue to function although the other muscles of respiration will be paralysed.

The upper limbs are innervated by the fifth cervical to the first thoracic segments via the brachial plexus.

Since the cervical spinal nerves are named after the vertebral body directly below them and the thoracic spinal nerves after the body immediately above them, there must be one more cervical spinal nerve than vertebra, i.e. there are eight cervical spinal nerves but only seven cervical vertebrae.

Fracture of the odontoid process

The odontoid process of the axis is enclosed by the anterior arch of the atlas and the transverse ligament of the atlas. It usually fractures at its base and, if the injury is not fatal, usually unites after a period of immobilization. However, non-union is not uncommon and some surgeons recommend grafting which has to be carried out through the back of the pharynx. Other surgeons prefer to reduce the fracture and then carry out a posterior spinal fusion from the skull to the second or third cervical vertebra.

Wedge fractures of cervical vertebral bodies

These fractures occur in flexion injuries but are relatively rare in comparison to those occurring in the thoracic or lumbar spine. They are usually stable and treatment in a supporting collar is adequate.

Dislocations of the cervical spine

As mentioned earlier, the inclination of the cervical articular facets makes them prone to dislocate in flexion injuries, e.g. falls on to the back of the head.

Depending on the size and direction of the force, either one or both facets become dislocated (Fig. 15.3). Damage to the cord may occur and pain down the limb due to root irritation is common. Fracture of the body or articular mass may occur.

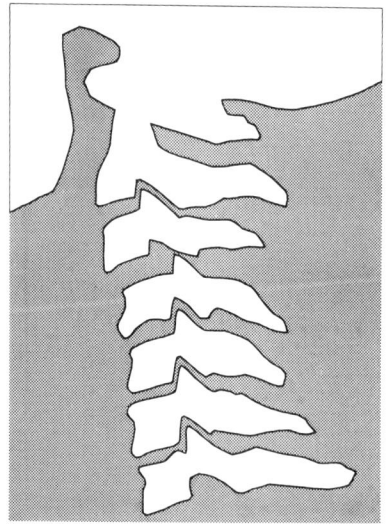

FIG. 15.3. A C3 on C4 dislocation of the cervical spine. Only one facet is dislocated.

Treatment

Reduction of the dislocation is usually achieved by applying traction to the cervical spine using skull calipers. The amount of traction is gradually increased under X-ray control until the facets are separated and unlocked and the traction then gradually diminished allowing the facets to 'seat home' again.

Post-operative immobilization firstly by traction and then by collar is continued for some months.

Some authorities prefer manipulative reduction under general anaesthesia with the use of relaxants.

Cervical spine dislocations in children
The cervical spines of children show a remarkably wide range of movement and are often mistakenly thought to have been dislocated. However, there is a definite danger of dislocation in children who have recently had a throat infection. In fact, spontaneous dislocation is not uncommon. Neurological complications are rare. Treatment consists of reduction by traction and immobilization until the capsular ligaments have returned to normal and the spine has become stable again.

Extension injuries of the cervical spine
A sudden extension of the cervical spine may strain the anterior longitudinal ligament and may also cause a fracture to the spinous process or the neural arch of a cervical vertebra. This type of injury is commonly seen nowadays in motorists whose cars are run into from behind while stationary. The hyperextension injury is usually followed by a flexion injury as the head comes forwards again.

The patient may have pain in the neck or down the arms and radiographs may show the fractures. Cervical traction may be necessary in severe injuries but collar immobilization is usually sufficient. The pain and stiffness may persist for many months.

DAMAGE TO THE SPINAL CORD

In all injuries to the vertebral column there is always the danger of damage to the spinal cord. This damage may be in the form of contusion, interference with blood-supply, or transection (partial or complete).

In the cervical region the nerve roots pass virtually horizontally out to the intervertebral foramina so that the problem of damage to the cord with sparing of the roots does not occur as it does in the lumbar region.

It is important for the surgeon to be able to assess the cord damage accurately in injuries in the cervical spine.

The problem is made more difficult because of the phenomenon of 'spinal shock'. By this is meant the virtual complete cessation of activity in the cord below the level of the lesion. The distinction between spinal shock and a complete transection of the cord may be difficult, but usually after complete transection localized reflex activity below the level of the lesion returns quite soon.

If therefore the patient with a cervical spine lesion is unable to move any of his limbs (tetraplegia) but reflex activity, e.g. ankle jerks, cremasteric reflex, or anal skin reflex, has returned it is highly likely that a complete transection has occurred.

The early management of a patient with a tetraplegia or paraplegia is directed towards keeping the skin intact and preventing distention and infection of the bladder. It will be dealt with more fully in Chapter 17.

The central cord syndrome
In some patients recovery from a tetraplegia is unusual in that the patient

regains the use of his legs but his upper limbs remain paralysed. This is explained as a form of ischaemic degeneration of the cervical spinal cord occurring in the area around the central canal. The ischaemia affects the long tracts from the upper limbs but spares those of the lower limbs. This is referred to as the central cord syndrome.

RECOMMENDATIONS FOR FURTHER READING

BURKE, D. C. and BERRYMAN, D. (1971) The place of closed manipulation in flexion–rotation dislocations of the cervical spine, *J. Bone Jt Surg.* **53B**, 165–81.

SIMMONS, E. H., BHALLA, S. K. and BUTT, W. P. (1969) Anterior cervical discectomy and fusion with a note on discography: technique and interpretation of results, *J. Bone Jt Surg.* **51B**, 225–37.

16 The thoracic spine

We shall discuss Scheurmann's disease and scoliosis under this section. Although it is true that all spinal conditions can affect any part of the spine, the main effects of these two conditions are seen in the thoracic area.

SCHEUERMANN'S DISEASE

In the early 1900s Scheuermann drew attention to a condition which causes an increase in the normal kyphosis of the thoracic spine—sometimes referred to as 'round back'. It is a disease of adolescents and is not usually painful.

Clinically the child is found to have an increase in the thoracic curve and tends to stand with the shoulders dropped forwards. Radiographs show some disorganization and fragmentation of the epiphysial areas of ossification at the upper and lower ends of the vertebral bodies.

Treatment consists of exercises designed to encourage 'arching' of the back and occasionally the use of a full-length back support (posterior spinal support). Vigorous flexion of the spine should be avoided.

The condition resolves when growth of the vertebral bodies is complete by which time treatment may have minimized the deformity.

SCOLIOSIS

Scoliosis may be defined as a lateral curvature of the spine. Most scoliotic spines have, in addition to the curvature, a rotatory deformity, the vertebral bodies being rotated towards the convex side of the curve.

Two main classifications are used, the first based on aetiology and the second on age of onset—the latter classification has a definite correlation with prognosis.

The aetiological classification

1. *Osteopathic.* In this type the causative abnormality is in the bony parts of the spine. They may be congenitally deformed or deformed by disease or trauma.
2. *Neuropathic.* The deformity is caused by muscle imbalance secondary to a neurological lesion. The common examples are poliomyelitis and cerebral palsy.
3. *Myopathic.* The underlying disease in this group is in the muscles themselves—myopathies.
4. *Idiopathic.* In this group the deformity apparently 'comes of itself', no demonstrable cause having been found. This constitutes by far the largest group.

The 'age-of-onset' classification

1. *Congenital.* The group consists of those cases in which there is a congenital anomaly in the spine.
2. *Infantile.* In these cases the curve becomes visible with the first 3 years of life. Most of them are of the idiopathic type but a congenital anomaly (osteopathic type) may first present at this time. The prognosis in the infantile idiopathic group is good—most cases resolve either spontaneously or on conservative treatment.
3. *Juvenile.* The curve appears at 4–9 years. Again, most of these cases are of the idiopathic type.
4. *Adolescent.* The curve appears after the age of 10 and before skeletal maturity is reached. These are the cases in which the prognosis is difficult to assess. Many cases get rapidly worse. These cases are usually of the idiopathic type, are commoner in girls than boys, and are usually convex to the right.

In practice we tend to use a combination of the above classifications, giving both the time of onset and the aetiology, e.g. adolescent idiopathic.

Symptoms

The patient, or the parents, are usually most concerned about the appearance of the back. It is very rare for scoliosis to cause discomfort before middle-age.

Signs

The curve may occur at any level.

1. Cervical and cervico-thoracic curves often cause a 'torticollis-type' deformity which may be associated with elevation of one shoulder.
2. Thoracic curves are the most common. The rotatory element of the deformity causes distortion of the chest cage, the ribs on the convex side being more prominent posteriorly. The resulting prominence or 'rib hump' can be made more obvious by getting the patient to bend forward (Fig. 16.1).
3. Thoraco-lumbar and lumbar curves tend to shift the upper part of the body over to one side relative to the pelvis, especially if the curve is not associated with a compensatory curve above it in the thoracic region. This offset makes the iliac crest more prominent on one side and the patient complains that 'one hip sticks out'.

The clinical examination should also elicit whether the curve is mobile, i.e. can be straightened by traction or flexion, or fixed, i.e. cannot be straightened. The two terms 'postural' and 'structural' are used by some surgeons to denote 'mobile' and 'fixed'.

It should be noted that any condition that causes tilting of the pelvis, e.g. inequality of leg length or an old dislocation of the hip will cause a compensatory scoliosis of the spine.

Effects of scoliosis

A curve of any marked degree of severity will reduce the vertical height of the patient.

The deformity of the chest cage will interfere with lung function, especially if the curve is more than 30°. Severe interference with pulmonary efficiency may lead to cor pulmonale. Patients with severely deformed chests are more prone to recurrent chest infections.

The thoracic spine 103

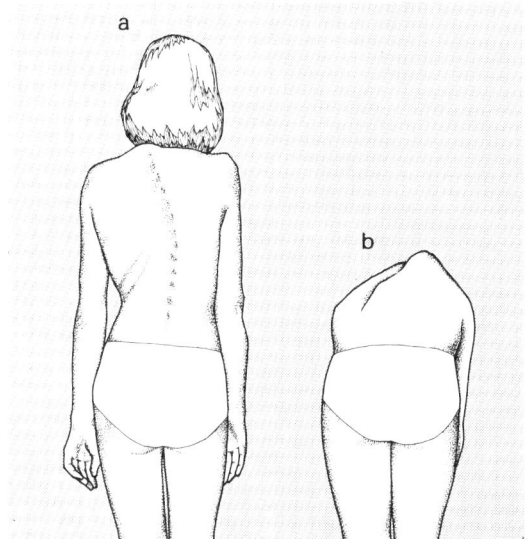

FIG. 16.1. Scoliosis of the spine. (a) Erect. (b) Bending forward.

Gross curves may distort the spinal canal and lead to traction on the spinal cord. This may lead to paraparesis or even paraplegia.

Measurement of scoliotic curves

An antero-posterior radiograph is taken of the spine. A line is drawn along the upper surface of the upper vertebra of the curve and another along the lower border of the lower vertebra of the curve. These lines are then produced until they meet and the angle between them measured. This is the Lippman–Cobb method of measurement and gives a result in degrees. It is sometimes difficult to identify the upper and lower borders of the vertebral bodies, especially in young children and those with anomalous vertebrae. The upper and lower limits of the curve are identified by tracing the curve upwards and downwards from the apex of the curve and identifying the first intervertebral disc space in which the two sides of the space are of equal height or the concave side is taller than the convex, i.e. the disc space at the level at which the curve either flattens out or changes over to a compensatory curve.

Treatment

The object of treatment is to end up with the smallest degree of deformity possible when the child has stopped growing. Although some progression of the curve may occur after growth of the spine has ceased, it is usually not of a significant degree.

Conservative treatment

Once the diagnosis of scoliosis has been made, it is important to keep the child under observation until growth ceases. She (or he) should be examined and the spine X-rayed periodically—the frequency of examination depending on the behaviour of the curve.

We use Risser's sign to estimate completion of spine growth. He pointed out that the centre of ossification for the iliac crest appears during the last 1–2 years of spinal growth, and by the time the ossification process has spread back as far as the posterior superior iliac spine, growth of the spine is complete.

Most of the work with scoliotic patients is in the form of periodic checks. It has been found that many curves can be prevented from deteriorating by conservative measures: remedial exercises and the wearing of the Milwaukee brace. This is a corset which is well supported by the pelvis and has an extension upwards to a head support. This tends to take the weight of the head off the spine and also, by means of a pad which is fixed to the support and presses on the rib hump, exert a gentle corrective force to the spine via the ribs.

Operative treatment
If it is found that the curve is becoming progressively worse in spite of conservative treatment, operative treatment is undertaken.

The standby of operative treatment is the posterior spinal fusion. This is usually done by removing the articular cartilage and underlying cortical bone from the posterior spinal articulations and placing bone grafts in the resulting spaces. Bone grafts are also placed on the laminae and spinous processes after decortication. The spine is then held in the position of maximum correction either by plaster of Paris body casts or by internal fixation using plates or rods, until the fusion is sound. By using the Roaf plate, correction of both the lateral curvature and the rotational deformity is obtained.

Other operative procedures include destruction of the growth areas of the bodies of the vertebrae on the convex side of the curve (epiphyseodesis) and cosmetic procedures such as removal of the blade of a prominent scapula or removal of unsightly bulges in the rib cage.

Recently it has been shown that the growth of the spine can be influenced by holding the ribs together on the convex side of the curve. This is done either by fusing the ribs or by 'binding' them with tapes. Results are encouraging.

Results. It must be realized that we are dealing here with a potentially progressive deformity, so that if a curve can be kept from progressing this can be considered a successful result. Some very gratifying corrections are obtained but some cases progress even after repeated operations.

RECOMMENDATIONS FOR FURTHER READING

JAMES, J. I. P. (1967) *Scoliosis*, E. & S. Livingstone, Edinburgh.
MOE, J. H. and KETTLESON, D. N. (1970) Idiopathic scoliosis, *J. Bone Jt Surg.* **52A**, 1509–33.
ROAF, R. (1966) *Scoliosis*, E. & S. Livingstone, Edinburgh.

17 The lumbar spine

ANATOMY

There are normally five lumbar vertebrae but some degree of fusion of the fifth lumbar vertebra to the first sacral vertebra is not uncommon. This is called 'sacralization' and is probably unimportant if the fusion—or lack of segmentation—affects both sides of the vertebra equally. Occasionally, however, the sacralization occurs on one side only and in these cases it is thought that the anomaly does predispose to backache.

The articular facets in the lumbar region lie in the sagittal plane and hence very little rotation can occur in this part of the spine. However, flexion and extension take place mainly at these joints.

The transverse processes in the lumbar region are large and give attachment to powerful muscles. They are very prone to fracture.

SPINA BIFIDA

The neural arches of the vertebrae are formed in the embryo from mesoderm which grows between the neural tube and the ectoderm. The neural tube, you will remember, is itself formed as an invagination of ectoderm which then loses its contact with the parent tissue.

If this development is upset, some gap may persist in the mesodermal tissues and their derivatives. This can vary from a small gap in the spinous process—spina bifida occulta—to a complete failure of the formation of the neural tube so that nerve tissue is present on the surface—myelomeningocoele. Occasionally an intermediate stage occurs in which the nerve tissue is covered by skin but the meninges are present under the skin as a fluctuant swelling—meningocoele.

The degree of neurological deficit in the lower limbs and the degree of control of the bowel and bladder sphincters varies according to the severity of the defect. In the most severe type there is complete paralysis of the lower limbs, with the exception of hip flexion, and loss of bowel and bladder control.

The orthopaedic surgeon's main aim is to stop the hips from dislocating due to uneven muscle action and to assist the child to walk by splintage or muscle-balancing operations. The main problems of treatment of these children are associated with urinary function and the prevention of urinary infections.

INFECTIONS OF THE LUMBAR SPINE

Tuberculous spondylitis has been discussed in Chapter 8 (p. 41). In practice, however, other bacteria are found to cause spondylitis more often than TB. Coliform infection is common in patients with urinary tract infections and staphylococcal infections of the discs and surrounding bone are not uncommon in children. They respond well to treatment with the appropriate antibiotic and bed rest.

BACKACHE AND SCIATIC NEURALGIA

The clinical approach to patients presenting at the clinic with backache and pain down the leg is virtually the same as in those with neckache and brachial neuralgia. A careful history is taken and the patient examined in order to decide which of the following three categories he or she falls into:

Category 1. Patients with backache only.
Category 2. Patients with backache plus sciatic neuralgia (sciatica).
Category 3. Patients with backache plus sciatica plus a neurological deficit in the lower limbs.

It is important to enquire whether the symptoms started after any particular activity or injury. Prolapse of the lower lumbar discs is very common and usually occurs while the patient is lifting a heavy weight.

In addition to checking the range of movement of the back, whether movement of the lumbar spine aggravates or brings on the pain, and whether there is any neurological deficit in the lower limbs, the following investigations are carried out:
1. A full examination of the abdomen with rectal examination if relevant.
2. The straight-leg raising test.

The straight-leg raising test
The patient lies supine on the couch. The examiner raises the non-painful leg, keeping the knee straight. In the normal patient the leg can be raised to 80° or 90° without more than slight tightness being felt behind the knee.

In a positive straight-leg raising test the range is diminished. The patient complains of pain down the back of the leg. This pain is aggravated by dorsiflexing the foot while holding the leg in the painful position. The pain is relieved by bending the knee. This all suggests that the sciatic nerve is sensitive to stretching. It should be emphasized that all three elements of the test should be positive before too much reliance is placed on it.

If the patient has a positive straight-leg raising test and is in Category 3, we can be reasonably certain that he or she has entrapment of the roots of the sciatic nerve. The cause of the entrapment varies according to the age of the patient.

Prolapse of the intervertebral disc

The intervertebral discs consist of a dense ring of fibrous tissue (annulus fibrosis) surrounding a soft fluid centre (nucleus pulposis). When subjected to heavy pressure the annulus may bulge and press on structures in the vicinity. If it bulges out on the anterior aspect of the spine it does not cause any symptoms. The evidence of previous anterior bulges are the 'osteophytes' on either side of the disc space which may be seen years later in the lateral radiograph.

If, however, the disc bulges or prolapses backwards, it protrudes into the spinal canal and may press on the cauda equina or a nerve root as it passes

The lumbar spine 107

downwards towards its intervertebral foramen. In these cases it may cause pain which will be felt in the distribution of that nerve root and weakness in the muscles supplied by it. Some numbness over the relevant dermatome may also be caused. If the prolapsed disc presses on the cauda equina it may cause loss of bladder control with consequent retention of urine.

Clinical features

If the fifth lumbar root is compressed the patient will complain of pain, mainly down the outer side of the calf and leg and the dorsum of his foot. He may have weakness of dorsiflexion of his toes and foot. The power of extension of the big toe is particularly suitable for testing and comparison with the normal side. Sensation to pinprick is usually reduced on the outer side of the calf and dorsum of the foot. The ankle jerk is usually diminished or absent.

If the first sacral root is compressed the pain will be in the calf, plantar flexion of the foot will be weak, there will be sensory blunting on the sole of the foot and up the back of the calf, and again the ankle jerk will be diminished or absent.

A central protrusion will cause difficulty with starting micturition or retention of urine, and there may be sensory blunting in the sacral segments (the 'saddle' area). It is important to test the saddle area in any patient with back symptoms, because this blunting of sensation is the only elicitable sign of compression of the lower sacral roots, their motor innervation being difficult to assess. Omission of this simple test may cause failure to diagnose cauda equina compression both in disc protrusions and in tumours.

Treatment

The vast majority of patients suffering from a prolapsed intervertebral disc will respond to conservative treatment. The regime prescribed depends partly on the personality of the patient and partly on the severity of the symptoms. Mild cases respond well to a short course of short-wave diathermy to the lumbar spine, and back extension exercises. More severe cases may require a period of a few months in an immobilizing corset. The surgical corset usually prescribed is reinforced with a rectangle of steel in the lumbar region and named after Dr. Goldthwait.

Very severe cases, and those who have not responded to the above treatments are admitted to the orthopaedic ward for a period of traction. This requires the patient to be in bed with the foot of the bed elevated and traction applied either to the pelvis using a corset, or to the legs using sticking-plaster strips applied to the sides of the legs and held on with an elasticated bandage.

With traction the pain usually settles in 7–10 days and the patient is then gradually mobilized wearing his Goldthwait support. We feel that it is unwise to maintain leg traction for more than 12–14 days because of the danger of thrombosis in the leg veins.

In a very small minority of patients the backache and sciatica persist even after 2 weeks on traction. If it is considered that he is still suffering from a prolapsed intervertebral disc (tumours and hysteria being another two causes of failure of traction) the patient is then investigated further by myelography preparatory to surgical exploration.

Myelogram. In this procedure a few millilitres of radio-opaque material are injected into the subarachnoid space and the shape of the dural theca inspected by positioning the patient in various postures and watching the movement of the dye on an X-ray image-intensification screen. A prolapsed intervertebral disc shows up as a negative dent in the dye column opposite a disc space.

Operative treatment. The indications for operation on a prolapsed intervertebral joint are therefore:
(1) failure of conservative treatment; or
(2) interference with bladder function in a central disc prolapse.
The latter is an indication for an emergency operation.

The spinal canal is opened from the back by removing part of the lamina (hence the name laminectomy) or, on occasion by just excising the ligamentum flavum (fenestration). The dura is then retracted and the prolapsed part of the disc identified, separated from the nerve root, and excised. It is customary to remove as much of the disc as possible in addition to the prolapsed position. Post-operatively the patient is kept in bed for 2 weeks and then allowed to mobilize wearing a support.

If strict criteria for operation are observed the success rate is high. If the operation is performed for less specific indications (e.g. on category 1 or 2 cases (p. 106)) the success rate is lower.

It is important to note that most cases of prolapse of the intervertebral discs occur in patients under the age of 50 years.

Lumbar spondylosis

Degeneration of discs in the lumbar region is probably the commonest cause of backache. It affects both sexes and its incidence increases with age. Patients are usually in category 1 or 2 but if osteophyte formation is marked or there is a history of prolapse of discs, the patient may have a neurological deficit.

Clinical features
Most patients exhibit restriction of the movements of the lumbar spine and exacerbation of pain on moving. The pain is often felt over the sacro-iliac joint. The straight-leg raising test often causes pain in the back, i.e. it is negative.

Radiographs
In early cases these may show narrowing of disc spaces, easily ascertained using MacNab's sign: a line drawn along the inferior border of the vertebral body as seen on the lateral radiograph and projected backwards should pass above the superior articular process of the vertebra below. If it cuts the articular process, the disc space is narrowed.

In late cases there is marked peridiscal osteophyte formation.

Treatment
Short-wave diathermy and back extension exercises are helpful in early cases. A strong back support is probably more beneficial in older patients. Fusion of the spine is very rarely indicated.

Osteoarthrosis of the lumbar spine

This condition is very common in the elderly, and most often affects the posterior joints between the fifth lumbar and the first sacral vertebrae. Backache and referred sciatica are the usual symptoms and examination reveals a restricted and painful range of flexion.

X-rays show degeneration of the L5–S1 and often the L4–L5 posterior articulations. The patients are usually in categories 1 or 2 but encroachment on the intervertebral foramina may cause a neurological deficit.

Lumbar spondylosis often coexists and the principles of treatment are similar.

ANKYLOSING SPONDYLITIS

This is an idiopathic condition affecting the sacroiliac joints, the spines, and occasionally the hips of young men. It can affect women, but rarely does so.

Pathology
The inflammation usually starts in the sacro-iliac joints which may or may not be painful. It then spreads up the spine, affecting the posterior joints and later the disc joints. As the disease progresses the joints gradually stiffen and are eventually replaced by bone. The final result is therefore a spine which is completely rigid. The course of the disease may take several years and tends to consist of relapses and remissions.

The hip joints, when involved, become stiff and painful and pass through a stage indistinguishable from primary osteoarthrosis before going on to bony fusion.

Aetiology
No cause has yet been found for this condition. Recent advances in tissue-typing techniques, developed for renal transplantation, have allowed researchers to investigate the tissue groups of these patients and a significant number of them (over 70 per cent) are found to belong to the same group, HLA 27.

Special investigations
The erythrocyte sedimentation rate is usually raised in acute episodes. The rheumatoid agglutination tests may be positive. Tissue typing may help in the diagnosis but the result is suggestive not diagnostic.

Radiographs
The earliest sign is loss of definition of the sacro-iliac joints. The hip joints

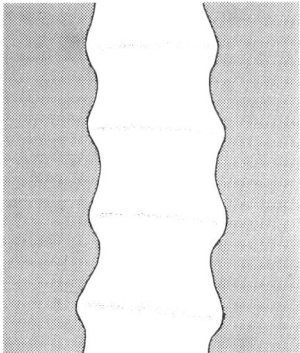

FIG. 17.1. The radiographic appearance of the lumbar spine affected with ankylosing spondylitis: the 'bamboo spine'.

may show the radiological features of osteoarthrosis. The final picture is of bony fusion of the sacro-iliac joints and occasionally the hip joints. The spine presents a classical picture of bony replacement of the disc spaces and posterior joints: the bamboo spine (Fig. 17.1).

Treatment
The philosophy of treatment is that we accept that the final stiffening of the spine is inevitable and therefore aim at keeping it in the optimum position.

The patient is assessed 3-monthly or 6-monthly and a measurement made of his spine. This can be done either by taking clinical photographs or by direct measurement using a spondylogram—a mechanical device which outlines the curve.

The natural tendency is for the spine to flex gradually because the patient either lies in bed with his head and shoulders propped up on pillows, or sits in an armchair in the flexed position.

If assessment shows that the spine has a tendency to flexion the patient is encouraged to sleep in the prone position or to lie supine on a hard bed without pillows. In this way we aim to have the spine stiffening in the anatomical position.

Pain is treated with analgesics. Some authorities use deep X-ray therapy if the pain is severe, but great care must be taken with dosage because of the danger of transverse myelitis and the production of malignant changes, especially in the marrow cells.

If the patient is first seen with marked flexion deformity of the spine (some patients cannot see the horizon) corrective osteotomy of the spine may be indicated.

Recently some patients with ankylosed hips have been treated by total hip replacement arthroplasty. The initial results are encouraging but there is, of course, a high probability that stiffening will recur.

TRAUMATIC LESIONS OF THE LUMBAR SPINE

Fractures of the transverse processes
These commonly occur either from direct injury or from sudden muscle pull. It should be remembered that there is a separate centre of ossification for the tip of the transverse process and fusion of this centre with the rest of the process may not occur.

These fractures virtually always unite without requiring any special treatment. The possibility of retro-peritoneal haemorrhage with resultant paralytic ileus must be kept in mind and the patient observed for 48 hours before being discharged.

Wedge fractures of the vertebral bodies
In normal individuals these fractures are caused by flexion strains and are often seen when the patient falls from a height onto his feet. The well-known triad of fractures of the calcaneum, crush fracture of a lumbar vertebra, and fracture of the upper cervical spine, should be looked for in any patient who has fallen from a height on to his feet. Crush or wedge fractures of the vertebral bodies are also common in patients suffering from osteoporosis.

These fractures are usually stable to flexion, extension, and rotation strains and can be treated by immobilization in bed until they are painless. The patient is then gradually mobilized in a back support and can return to his occupation when the fracture has consolidated.

The old practice of immobilizing these patients in a plaster of Paris body cast in extension has not been shown to improve the results of treatment and so has been largely abandoned.

Some degree of abdominal distension and ileus is again common following these fractures.

Fracture dislocations of the spine

The shape of the articular processes and the plane of the posterior joints make pure dislocation of the lumbar spine almost impossible.

The stablity of the spine to flexion–extension and rotational strains depends on the integrity of both the vertebral body-disc anterior joint and the posterior joint and its ligaments, which are reinforced by the interspinous and supraspinous ligaments.

The common injury which causes an unstable fracture dislocation is a combination of a flexion strain and a rotation strain. This usually affects the junctional area between the flexible lumbar spine and the mobile thoracic spine, i.e. the twelfth thoracic and first and second lumbar vertebrae. The injury is commonly produced when a heavy weight falls onto a workman who is bending forwards (e.g. a miner in a fall of rock), or when the patient falls from a height onto the back and shoulders (e.g. a steeplechase jockey who is thrown at a jump).

The injury consists usually of a fracture through the articular processes and a horizontal fracture across the body of the vertebra. The name 'slice fracture' is given to this fracture. Following it, the spine in this area is unstable to flexion-extension and rotation strains and damage to the contents of the spinal canal is common, i.e. there is a high risk of paraplegia.

Treatment of the fracture
If there is no neurological damage and the patient has normal sensation in the back, buttocks, and thighs, he can be treated on a plaster bed. Non-union of the fracture is rare.

If there is a sensory deficit on the back buttocks or thighs, the patient must not be left lying on these areas but must be turned from side to side every 4 hours. There are two schools of thought as to the treatment of the fracture in these circumstances:
1. The Stoke Mandeville school feel that the spine should not be fixed but that a team of nurses should be specially trained in the art of turning the patient without displacing the fracture.
2. The Sheffield school feel that the fracture should be immobilized by the insertion of a plate fixed to the spinous processes above and below the fracture because this facilitates the turning of the patient and prevents further damage to the contents of the spinal canal.

The treatment of paraplegia
Immediately following the injury there will be a period of spinal shock. As in

the case of the cervical spine, return of reflex movement without voluntary control strongly suggests transection of the cord.

You will notice that in this section on the lumbar spine the expression 'contents of the spinal canal' has been used rather than 'spinal cord'. This is because the situation at the level of the upper lumbar spine is a little more complicated than in that in the cervical spine.

At the level of the upper border of the first lumbar vertebra, the spinal canal contains:

1. The spinal cord—the lumbosacral junction of cord segments (L5–S1) lies at the level of the thoracolumbar junction in the vertebral column (T12–L1).
2. The nerve roots of the spinal nerves from the second lumbar downwards. This is because the spinal cord has not kept pace with the vertebral column during growth and when maturity is reached the lower end of the spinal cord lies opposite the second lumbar vertebra. The rest of the spinal canal below this is therefore occupied by nerve roots passing down to reach their respective intervertebral and sacral foramina.

An injury at the common level of the thoracolumbar junction of the vertebral column may therefore:

(1) transect the cord and the nerve roots, causing complete paralysis below L2;
(2) transect the cord but not damage the roots, causing paralysis below S1; this phenomenon is referred to as 'root escape';
(3) do varying degrees of damage to both cord and roots;
(4) do no permanent damage to either cord or roots.

Remember that regeneration may occur in roots but not in the cord. Remember also that the spinal centre for bladder control is at the level of the third sacral segment.

The initial treatment. The efficacy of early treatment of paraplegia depends on a full appreciation of the disadvantages under which the patient is placed. These are two:

1. Loss of skin sensation means that the patient has no warning that a particular area of skin has been rendered ischaemic by pressure. Normally we are subconsciously aware of this phenomenon and move about to 'get comfortable'. For this reason the patient must not be allowed to lie in one position for more than 2 hours but moved, e.g. from side to side, or side to back, at regular intervals. If this is not done the skin and subcutaneous tissue become necrotic and a pressure sore results. After a few days this period can safely be extended to 4 hours.

2. Loss of bladder innervation means that he has neither the sensation of fullness of his bladder nor the ability to void. If left untreated his bladder will distend to its maximum and then dribble incontinently (overflow incontinence). The distention may cause permanent paralysis of the bladder musculature. The use of an indwelling catheter is to be deprecated as this rapidly introduces infection. The treatment of the bladder in paraplegia adopted in our orthopaedic unit therefore is to prevent distention by intermittent catheterization (either 8- or 12-hourly depending on the patients intake of fluid), specimens being taken regularly for bacteriological study. In this way infection can usually be prevented for 2–3 weeks. It must be emphasized that this catheterization must be carried out with full aseptic precautions.

Long-term treatment of paraplegia. This is usually carried out in special units and consists of:
1. Rehabilitation of the patient as an individual.
2. The learning of new methods of locomotion, either with crutches, sticks, or wheelchair, depending on the severity of the paralysis.
3. The learning of methods of bladder control. Completely paralysed bladders often regain the facility of reflex emptying and patients learn various methods of initiating these reflexes, e.g. pinching the inner side of the thigh. The wearing of some form of collecting device is, however, usually necessary.
4. Learning to protect the integrity of the skin by periodically relieving weight bearing.
5. Learning to control bowel actions by means of suppositories or enemas.

Many paraplegic patients are now returned to a very useful place in society.

Spondylolysis

This term is used to denote the condition in which there is loss of bony continuity of the neural arch of a vertebra. The condition may be painless or may cause backache with or without sciatic neuralgia. It does not cause a neurological deficit in the lower limbs, i.e. the patients are in categories 1 and 2 (p. 106).

Characteristically the 'gap' or loss of continuity occurs at the junction of the pedicle in lamina if the vertebra is viewed from above and, if it is viewed from the side, in that part of the bone between the superior and inferior articular processes, i.e. the pars interarticularis. For this reason it is called a pars interarticularis defect (Fig. 17.2). It occurs most commonly in the fourth and the fifth lumbar vertebrae.

Radiograph

The defect may be visible in the lateral view but is more obvious in oblique views. In this view the outline of the lamina, superior and inferior articular processes, and the transverse process resemble the silhouette of a Scottish terrier, the pars interarticularis corresponding to the neck of the dog. A defect appears as a collar on the dog.

Treatment

The use of a back support of the Goldthwait type usually cures the symptoms. There is a small danger that the pars interarticularis may gradually 'give way' and follow-up radiography is advisable.

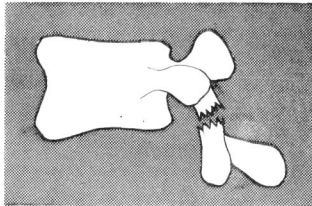

FIG. 17.2. Spondylolysis: a lateral view of the fifth lumbar vertebra showing the defect in the pars interarticularis.

114 *Orthopaedics for Undergraduates*

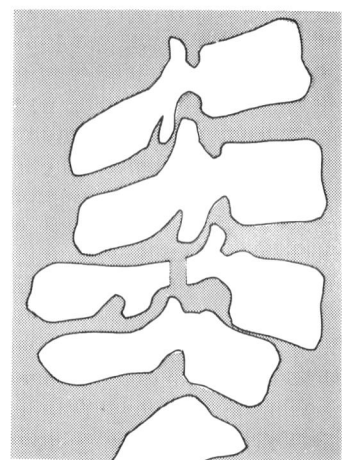

FIG. 17.3. Radiographic appearance of spondylolisthesis of the fourth lumbar vertebra on the fifth.

Spondylolisthesis

In this condition one vertebral body moves forward on the body below it. It may case backache or backache with sciatic neuralgia. Root compression may occur with resulting neurological deficit in the lower limbs, i.e. the patients may be in category 1, 2, or 3. The condition is commonest in the fifth lumbar vertebra, causing a forward shift of the vertebra on the sacrum, but also often seen in the fourth lumbar vertebra (Fig. 17.3).

Causes
There are three common causes of this condition:
1. Fractures of the neural arch.
2. Separation of the two parts of the neural arch in cases of spondylolysis.
3. Gross osteoarthrosis of the posterior joints with displacement of the upper vertebra. Occasionally in osteoarthrosis the opposite deformity occurs, i.e. the upper vertebra is displaced backwards on the vertebra below and to this phenomenon the name 'retrospondylolisthesis' is given.

Treatment
   1. In the traumatic type the treatment depends on the severity of the injury and the presence or absence of damage to the contents of the spinal canal (see p. 112).
   2. Separation of a spondylolytic neural arch is usually a gradual phenomenon, and reduction is not possible. Several degrees of displacement are described, depending on the extent of the 'travel' relative to the anteroposterior diameter of the vertebra below. Patients with minor degrees of slip are usually kept relatively symptom-free by wearing a strong support. More severe degrees of slip and those which do not respond to conservative treatment are usually treated by spinal fusion.
   3. Gross osteoarthrosis of the posterior joints is rendered painless in the vast majority of patients by the wearing of a support. Very rarely the condition may require fusion.

RECOMMENDATIONS FOR FURTHER READING

HOLDSWORTH, F. (1970) Fractures, dislocations and fracture-dislocations of the spine, *J. Bone St Surg.* **52A**, 1534–51.

RANG, M. (1966) Marie's original description of ankylosing spondylitis (Spondylosis Rhizomelique). In *Anthology of Orthopaedics*, pp. 120–5, E. & S. Livingstone, Edinburgh.

SHARRARD, W. J. W. (1971) Congenital and development abnormalities of the neuraxis. In *Paediatric Orthopaedics and Fractures*, Chapter 14, pp. 596–691, Blackwell, Oxford.

18 The pelvis and sacrum

CONDITIONS OF THE PELVIS

There are very few conditions that specifically affect the pelvis, but some of the conditions which also affect other parts of the skeleton deserve mention. These are Paget's disease and acute osteomyelitis and tuberculosis. The conditions peculiar to the pelvis which will be described are osteitis pubis and tears of the adductor origin.

Paget's disease of the pelvis

The pelvis is one of the bones which is commonly affected by Paget's disease. It may start in the ilium, ischium, or pubis and often affects all three. Coexistent Paget's disease of the femur is occasionally seen. The patient may have no symptoms from the disease or, on the other hand, may have some dull pain, usually felt in the buttock or in the iliac crest region. If, however, the disease affects the acetabulum, degenerative arthorosis may occur and this of course, may be painful.

The treatment of arthrosis of the hip secondary to Paget's disease does not at the moment differ from primary osteoarthrosis, but the underlying Paget's disease may be treated by medical means, e.g. by the administration of thyrocalcitonin or fluorides. Malignant change (osteosarcoma) of Paget's disease of the pelvis has been reported.

Acute osteomyelitis of the pelvis

This condition is singled out for special mention because of the difficulty with diagnosis. It occurs mainly in children and, if near the hip joint, may present as a septic arthritis with a painful irritable joint, high white cell count, and pyrexia. If there is any suggestion of involvement of the hip joint, early exploration and decompression should be carried out.

If the focus is not near the hip joint, it is best treated with the appropriate antibiotic after the preliminary taking of a blood sample for bacteriological culture.

Tuberculosis of the pelvis

Characteristically, tuberculosis affects the region of the sacro-iliac joints. Clinical features are often minimal, although slight aching and tenderness may be present.

Radiographs

These show areas of sclerosis and porosis lateral to the joint line which may itself be obscured. The main difficulty is in distinguishing the condition from three other conditions with similar radiographic changes:

(1) pyogenic osteomyelitis;
(2) ankylosing spondylitis;
(3) osteitis condensans ilii.

The white cell count and blood culture result should help to exclude the first. Other stigmata of ankylosing spondylitis should be looked for, e.g. stiffness of the spine and decrease in the degree of chest expansion. The third condition, osteitis condensans ilii, is a radiological diagnosis; no clinical features are associated with it.

Biopsy may be necessary to establish the diagnosis.

The treatment of tuberculosis of the sacro-iliac region follows the same principles as those for the condition when it occurs elsewhere in the spine.

Osteitis pubis

Inflammation of the pubis is rare, but it is most commonly seen following operations on the bladder and prostate gland. The patient usually complains of a dull ache in the pubic area some months after the operation.

Clinical examination reveals tenderness and warmth in this area and radiographs may show areas of sclerosis and/or bone destruction in the body of the pubis and the superior pubic ramus.

Most patients respond well to antibiotics, and surgical exploration is not usually necessary.

Tears of the adductor origin

Damage to the muscle fibres and periosteum of the inferior pubic ramus are commonly seen in individuals who fall with their hips abducted, e.g. footballers stretching to kick the ball when it is almost out of reach.

These patients have pain in the region of the inferior pubic ramus. The area may be tender to pressure and forcing abduction of the hip reproduces the pain.

Radiographs taken some weeks after the injury, or in patients suffering from recurrent symptoms, may show areas of new bone formation lateral to the inferior pubic ramus.

Symptoms usually subside with rest. Occasionally it is necessary to inject the area with hydrocortisone. This procedure usually relieves symptoms.

FRACTURES OF THE PELVIS

When discussing fractures, it is useful to consider the pelvis as a circular structure which acts as the connection between the spine and the two lower limbs and conducts the forces of weight bearing. The part of the pelvis which corresponds anatomically to the ring is the inlet of the true pelvis and the other parts of the pelvis, e.g. ischium or iliac crests, may be considered as appendages to the ring. The reason for this analogy is that if the 'ring' is broken at one point in its circumference it is likely that it is also disrupted at another point. Appreciation of this fact helps us to avoid overlooking secondary and less obvious disruptions.

In addition to the fractures of the pelvic ring and isolated 'appendage' fractures, we must also consider fractures of the base of the acetabulum which range from undisplaced cracks to total 'stove-in pelvis' injuries and are described in Chapter 25 (on the hip joint).

The classification of fractures of the pelvis therefore is into:
(1) isolated fractures of ilium, ischium, and pubis;
(2) compression fractures of the pubis;
(3) fractures of the pelvic ring;
(4) fractures of the acetabulum.

Isolated fractures of the pelvis

These are usually due to direct violence or, occasionally, to sudden muscle contraction: the anterior inferior iliac spine may be avulsed in footballers, especially during adolescence. The commoner isolated fractures are those of the inferior pubic ramus or the iliac crest. Since the integrity of the pelvic ring is preserved these fractures are best treated by early movement and weight bearing.

Compression fractures of the pubis

Antero-posterior compression of the pelvis may result in fractures of all four pubic rami. The degree of displacement is usually slight so that reduction is not usually required. The rate of union is high.

There is a danger of damage to the genito-urinary tract with these fractures. This is described later.

Fractures of the pelvic ring

These are seen following industrial and road traffic injuries. The common type is a fracture through both pubic rami on one side with either a vertical fracture through the ilium from crest to sciatic notch or a disruption of the sacro-iliac joint. The two breaks in the ring tend to occur diagonally opposite each other, e.g. pubic rami on the left and sacro-iliac joint on the right (Fig. 18.1). Manipulative reduction by pulling on the lower limb with the patient under general anaesthesia may be necessary. It is important to realize that if the patient is allowed to walk before these injuries have consolidated, they will be subjected to shearing strains and delayed union may occur. Patients who have

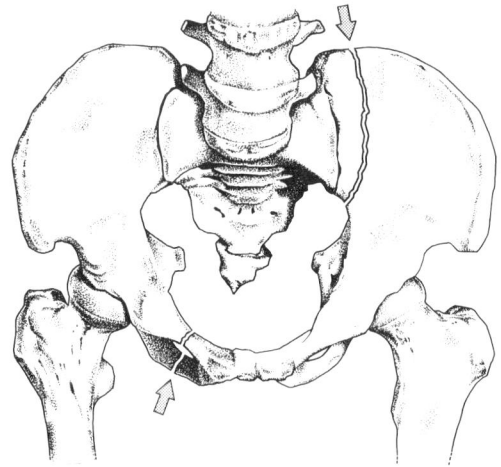

FIG. 18.1. Double fracture of the pelvic ring.

sustained double disruptions of the pelvic ring are therefore kept in bed, with leg traction, until the fractures have united.

Oystering of the pelvis
A variation of the pelvic-ring disruption is occasionally seen in patients whose injuries have been such that the pubic bones have been fractured or the symphysis split and the two sides of the pelvis have been opened up like the covers of a book. There is often marked separation present anteriorly. These patients are treated in slings, which have the same effect as a hammock, namely, the two sides of the pelvis are closed together. Bilateral leg traction is also applied.

Complications of fractures of the pelvis

Haemorrhage
Bleeding from injuries to the pelvis may be profuse. The difficulty confronting the surgeon is that this bleeding may not be obvious. This is because the blood accumulates in the easily distensible areolar tissue between the peritoneum and the muscles of the posterior abdominal wall. It is not unusual for a patient with a fracture of the pelvis to lose 2 litres of blood into these tissues. For this reason it is important to have an intravenous infusion set up as soon as possible in any patient in this category. The first sign that the patient has lost a considerable quantity of blood may be a sudden and profound drop in blood-pressure.

It is also important to make a full examination of the patient's abdomen as early as possible in his assessment. This is because the retroperitoneal bleeding may cause the onset of paralytic ileus and the examiner may then be unable to decide whether the patient has sustained an intra-abdominal injury in addition to his pelvic fracture.

Damage to the genito-urinary tract
The lower parts of the ureters, the bladder and the urethra, are related very closely to the pelvis—indeed the urethra in the male passes through the perineal membrane which is stretched between the inferior pubic rami. Any sudden alteration in the shape of the pelvis may damage the lower genito-urinary tract, particularly the membranous urethra. In addition the object that damaged the pelvis, e.g. the wheel of the vehicle which ran over a patient, may also have damaged the bladder.

The presence of blood at the external urinary meatus is highly suggestive of damage to the genito-urinary tract.

Assessment. There are two schools of thought on this subject: the Bristol school feels that if there is any possibility of damage the patient should be examined in theatre using a urethroscope. This is recommended because in some cases of damage to the urethra there is a bridge of mucosa extending across the tear and its preservation is important as it contributes to the proper healing of the urethra.

The other school feels that early diagnosis of urethral damage is more important and recommends the passing of a fine catheter as soon as the condition of the patient allows. If the catheter passes into the bladder and clear urine drains out through the catheter it means that there is unlikely to be any damage to the genito-urinary tract. If the catheter passes into the bladder and blood-stained urine is drained, then some degree of damage has occurred but not sufficient to warrant emergency exploration. If it is impossible to pass a catheter, surgical exploration is necessary.

In all three instances, the catheter will probably be left in the bladder for a period because of the difficulty in micturition and the pain on straining.

In most departments the orthopaedic surgeon usually leaves the decision as to investigation and treatment of genito-urinary tract damage to the genito-urinary surgeon. Most units belong to the immediate-catheterization school.

CONDITIONS OF THE SACRUM AND COCCYX

Coccydynia

Pain in the coccygeal region is a distressing symptom that usually occurs in women. It commonly occurs following childbirth but is also seen after injuries when the patient falls onto the coccyx. The main symptom is pain on sitting, especially on a hard surface.

Rectal examination with the index finger in the rectum and the thumb on the posterior aspect of the coccyx may reveal tenderness of the coccyx itself or pain on moving the sacro-coccygeal joint.

Radiographs may show an abnormally long coccyx or acute anterior angulation of it.

Treatment

Most cases respond to an injection of hydrocortisone into the tender periosteum or joint. Very occasionally excision of the coccyx (coccygectomy) is necessary.

Fractures of the sacrum

Fractures of the sacrum are virtually always due to direct injury and they usually unite without undue delay.

The problems of these fractures arise if they involve the sacral foramina and cause damage to the sacral nerves. The main complications are sciatica if any of the upper three foramina are involved, and interference with bladder function if any of the second, third, or fourth foramina are involved.

Paralysis of bladder function tends to be temporary, suggesting neurapraxia rather than axonotmesis or neurotmesis. The management of the bladder is, of course, similar to that in injuries at higher levels in the vertebral column as discussed in Chapter 17 in the section on paraplegia (p. 111).

RECOMMENDATIONS FOR FURTHER READING

ALMOND, G. and VERNON, E. (1959) Iliac skeletal traction. A method of treatment of 'oyster-shell' pelvis, *J. Bone Jt Surg.* **41B**, 779–81.

PELTIER, L. F. (1965) Complications associated with fractures of the pelvis, *J. Bone Jt Surg.* **47A**, 1060–9.

19 The shoulder region

ANATOMY

The shoulder, or 'gleno-humeral' joint, is a ball-and-socket joint. The ball consists of the head of the humerus and the socket the glenoid fossa of the scapula. This bony socket is very shallow but it is made deeper by the fibro-cartilaginous rim called the glenoid labrum, around its periphery. This rim attaches both to the bony glenoid and to the capsule of the joint near its attachment to the glenoid.

The tendons of the muscles inserting into the greater and lesser tuberosities of the humerus tend to blend with each other and with the capsule of the shoulder joint forming a thick layer called the 'rotator cuff' of the shoulder joint. The muscles concerned are supra-spinatus, infra-spinatus, subscapularis, and teres minor.

Movements

The normal shoulder joint exhibits the following ranges of movement. Abduction: 0–90°; internal rotation 0–90°; external rotation 0–90°. When the arm is abducted to the vertical position, the first 90° of movement takes place at the gleno-humeral joint and the range from 90° to 180° takes place at the interface between the scapula and the chest wall.

CLINICAL CONDITIONS OF THE SHOULDER

Sprengel's shoulder

This is a congenital condition in which the scapula is smaller and higher than normal. It may affect both shoulders in one individual and the appearance in such a patient will be not unlike that of a patient with the Klippel–Feil syndrome, i.e. the patient appears to have no neck, as his head seems to come straight up from the chest (Fig. 19.1).

There is in addition to the abnormal scapula a second anomaly: in the majority of cases there is an abnormal bar of bone connecting the scapula to the vertebral column: the omovertebral bone.

The range of movement at the shoulder joint is usually normal but scapulo-thoracic movement may be limited.

Treatment

If the condition affects one shoulder, the cosmetic blemish may be severe and operative removal of the omovertebral bar and transposition of the scapula to a lower level is advisable. Bilateral cases and mild unilateral cases should be carefully assessed before advising correction.

The appearance may also be improved by removing parts of the vertebra which are prominent.

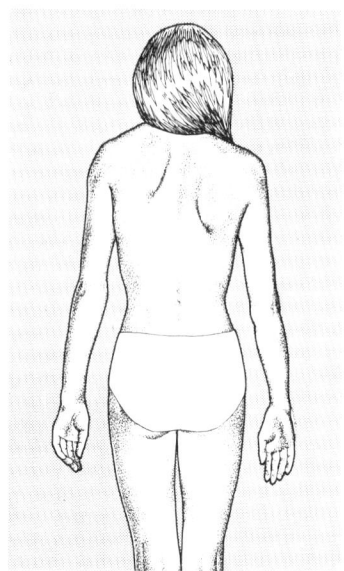

FIG. 19.1. Sprengel's shoulder.

Capsulitis (frozen shoulder)
This is a common condition affecting the middle-aged and elderly. It is characterized by pain and stiffness of the shoulder joint, and typically continues for many months and sometimes up to as long as a year.

Cause
In most cases no cause is found. In some cases the symptoms come on soon after a fall.

Symptoms
The patient notices some pain and restriction in the range of movement of the shoulder joint, characteristically noticing difficulty with tying of an apron or with combing the hair. Pain comes on usually slowly at first and is felt over the point of the shoulder or at the point of insertion of the deltoid muscle.

Signs
On examination, one finds a restriction of range of movement of the shoulder, particularly of internal rotation. There is also pain at the extremes of the range of movement. Radiographs are usually non-contributory.

Treatment
During the acutely painful stage rest is indicated. Short-wave diathermy may ease the pain. After the pain has begun to settle, movement is encouraged. If it is found that stiffness of the shoulder persists for some time after the pain has settled, manipulation of the shoulder under a general anaesthetic is indicated.

Results
Relief of pain occurs but may take several months. There is usually a return of a useful range of movement although the range may not be complete.

Prognosis
It is unlikely that the condition will recur on the same side but similar attacks affecting the other shoulder are quite common.

Supraspinatus tendinitis

This is an inflammatory condition usually localized to the upper part of the rotator cuff region of the capsule of the shoulder joint. The condition may progress to spontaneous rupture of the supraspinatus tendon. The condition is seen in middle-aged and elderly patients. The cause is unknown.

Pathology
An area of degeneration occurs usually about 1 cm from the insertion of the supraspinatus tendon. The area may degenerate into a cheese-like substance and may become calcified.

Symptoms
Acute pain is felt over the tip of the shoulder on abduction of the upper limb. The pain may not be felt as abduction is started but comes on during one part of the movement often disappearing as abduction approaches 180°. This is referred to as the 'painful arc syndrome' and is probably due to the inflamed area of tendon coming into contact with the acromion process.

Signs
Tenderness is usually present over the supraspinatus tendon area. Abduction of the shoulder is painful. There may be restriction of abduction and if rupture of the supraspinatus tendon has occurred there is the classical sign of elevation of that side of the shoulder girdle when the patient attempts to abduct the upper limb.

Radiographs
These may show calcification in the supraspinatus tendon, during or soon after the acute pain (Fig. 19.2).

Treatment
Some surgeons suggest needling or injection of local anaesthetic into the calcareous area in the tendon. This occasionally affords complete symptomatic relief. If the tendon has ruptured, operative repair is indicated although the results are not universally successful. At operation it is commonly found that the tear involves a large part of the rotator cuff.

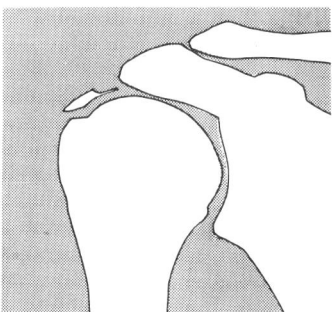

FIG. 19.2. Calcification in the supraspinatus tendon.

Rheumatoid disease
The shoulder joint is commonly affected in rheumatoid disease, but usually in association with other joints. Rotator cuff tears occur more commonly in patients with rheumatoid disease.

Osteoarthrosis
This is a rare affection of the shoulder joint but may be very disabling if the patient has osteoarthrosis of the lower limb joints as well because the shoulder degeneration makes the use of crutches very difficult.

INJURIES IN THE SHOULDER REGION

Fracture of the surgical neck of the humerus
This injury occurs in two main groups:
(1) In the young, the injury is usually associated with a separation of the epiphysis from the upper end of the humerus.
(2) In the elderly.

The injury usually follows a fall on the outstretched hand but may also occur after a fall onto the shoulder area. The patient finds that he or she is unable to abduct or flex the upper limb. Examination reveals bruising, swelling, and tenderness deep to the deltoid muscle and confirms the loss of power of shoulder movement.

Radiographs
In the elderly these may show a little angulation or displacement and occasionally the head of the humerus is rotated on the neck. This is seen particularly in comminuted fractures. In the young there may be a marked degree of displacement.

Treatment
1. In the young it must be remembered that a great deal of moulding can occur at the upper end of the humerus and a moderate degree of displacement can be accepted. If the head of the humerus has rotated into abduction the limb should be immobilized with the arm abducted 90°.
2. In the elderly, if the fracture is undisplaced, the patient is treated by immobilization in a collar-and-cuff sling or a full arm sling for 2–3 weeks. When the pain has passed off, mobilization of the shoulder is commenced.

Badly displaced fractures or fractures with rotation of the head may require open reduction, but internal fixation is only very occasionally indicated.

Fracture of the acromion
This injury is usually caused by forced abduction of the shoulder and it is usually an undisplaced fracture. It is treated by resting the arm in a full arm sling until the fracture has become painless. Active movement is then started.

Fracture of the greater tuberosity
This is usually associated with dislocation of the shoulder joint, and a reduction of the dislocation usually causes reduction of the fracture of the greater tuberosity. However, it may occur as an isolated injury, and if markedly displaced either as an isolated injury or after reduction of the dislocation of the shoulder, it should be reduced and internally fixed.

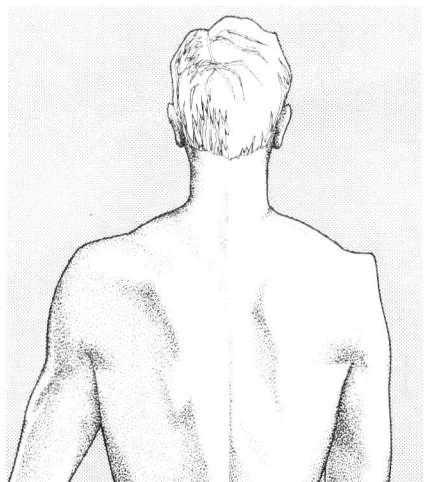

FIG. 19.3. The characteristic appearance of a dislocated shoulder viewed from behind.

Dislocation of the shoulder joint

This is a very common injury, rare in childhood but occurring at any age thereafter. It is usually caused by falling on the outstretched arm and is therefore a common Rugby football injury. There are two types:
1. The humeral head may displace anteriorly and come to lie below the coracoid process. This is the common type and is referred to as the sub-coracoid or anterior dislocation of the shoulder.
2. The humeral head may dislocate posteriorly (rare).

Symptoms

The patient complains of pain and an inability to move the shoulder joint.

Signs

The common anterior dislocation is best diagnosed by inspecting the patient from behind. The normal curved contour of the shoulder is replaced by an acute angle or cut-off appearance (Fig. 19.3). This is due to the fact that the greater tuberosity no longer holds out the deltoid muscle and this falls as a curtain from the outer edge of the acromion process. In a thin person the empty glenoid fossa can be felt and the bulge of the head of the humerus below the coracoid process may also be palpable. In an obese person the diagnosis may be difficult. In these cases Dugas' sign may be helpful. It is usually impossible to place the hand of the suspect limb on the front of the opposite shoulder in cases of dislocation of the shoulder, i.e. adduction and internal rotation are limited.

Radiographs

An antero-posterior view usually confirms anterior dislocation but a lateral view of the upper humerus and shoulder joint may be necessary to confirm posterior dislocation. The lateral radiograph is taken with the arm abducted 90° on the shoulder joint, the X-ray tube in the axilla and the X-ray plate resting on the top of the deltoid. The reason that this may be necessary in a posterior dislocation is that the head of the humerus does not sink down but stays at its normal level merely passing posteriorly out of the glenoid and the position may look normal on an antero-posterior X-ray.

Treatment
Reduction of a dislocated shoulder is indicated. Many methods are described. The method recommended is that the patient should be under a general anaesthetic with relaxants. Traction is then applied along the line of the limb with an assistant applying counter-traction to the thorax. The humeral head can usually be lifted over the inferior rim of the glenoid after traction has been applied for a few minutes.

If the patient is unsuitable for general anaesthesia, an attempt at the 'hanging-arm' method is recommended. The patient lies face downwards on the couch and the affected arm is allowed to hang over the side of the couch. Analgesic drugs are given and the muscles around the shoulder joint, which had been put into spasm by the dislocation, relax and allow the head of the humerus to pass around the inferior edge of the glenoid and reduction of the dislocation is achieved.

Following reduction of the dislocation it is important to immobilize the upper limb until the capsule has become re-attached to the edge of the glenoid and anterior surface of the scapula. In a young person this is particularly important. The arm is immobilized against the side of the chest with the elbow flexed about 110°. This is best achieved by applying a collar-and-cuff sling, placing a wad of cotton wool in the axilla, and strapping the arm to the side. In a young person this position should be maintained for 3 weeks. In the elderly some stiffness of the shoulder may result if the immobilization is continued for as long as this and after 7–10 days mobilization should be started. This period of immobilization in young people should be stressed because of the danger of recurrent dislocation of the shoulder if early mobilization is allowed.

Recurrent dislocation of the shoulder
This is a disabling condition usually found in young active men. In the vast majority of cases there is a history of a traumatic dislocation in the past. There is also a rare type of recurrent dislocation due to congenital laxity of the shoulder joint but this is seen in young children and the capsule usually tightens up with age so that the condition is self-curing.

Cause
In most cases of recurrent dislocation of the shoulder a history of acute traumatic dislocation is obtained and, if the patient is questioned carefully, in a large percentage of cases it will be realized that the immobilization following reduction of his original dislocation was of the order of 3–4 days or less.

Pathology
The attachment of the capsule to the front of the scapula and to the rim of the glenoid is interrupted. This allows the capsule to balloon forward, which in turn allows the humeral head to pass over the rim of the glenoid. The glenoid labrum usually retains it attachment to the capsule but the anterior part of its attachment to the glenoid is lost and the labrum becomes attenuated. The repeated contact of the back of the humeral head with the edge of the glenoid

may give rise to a groove in that part of the head of the humerus. This is referred to as the 'hatchet' deformity.

Symptoms

The patient usually gives a history of repeated dislocations of the shoulder, each dislocation occurring with a progressively smaller amount of force. In time the shoulder joint becomes very lax and may dislocate on very mild external rotation of the shoulder, e.g. on opening the newspaper. More sensitive patients may mention a feeling of insecurity in the shoulder and an apprehension because it feels as though it is going to dislocate.

Signs

Clinical examination is usually negative except in some patients the apprehension mentioned above may be experienced by the patient when the arm is fully externally rotated. Examination under general anaesthesia may prove the diagnosis, and in some cases the head is easily dislocated forwards.

Recurrent posterior dislocation of the humeral head is very rare but does occur.

Radiographs

Conventional X-rays are not usually helpful. The lateral view may show the 'hatchet' deformity.

Treatment

In the elderly, operative treatment is probably not indicated and the patient should instead be cautioned to limit the use of his shoulder. However, most patients suffering from this condition are young, healthy men often engaged in occupations such as scaffolding or building, and in these cases the recurrent dislocation of the shoulder is a severe disability. It is customary to define a recurrent dislocation as one which has occurred more than twice and occurs with diminishing amounts of force on each occasion.

Operative treatment. There are two main operations described and it is our practice to carry out a combination of both of these operations if the findings

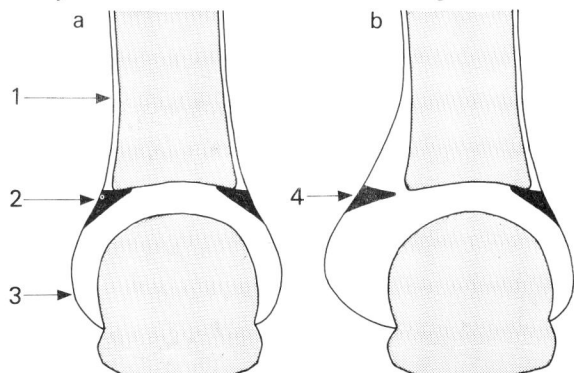

FIG. 19.4. Recurrent dislocation of the shoulder. (a) The normal shoulder viewed from above: (1) anterior surface of the scapula; (2) glenoid labrum; (3) capsule of the shoulder joint. (b) The findings in recurrent dislocation: (4) Bankart lesion.

warrant it. The shoulder is opened via an anterior approach and the labrum is identified and re-attached to the glenoid by means of catgut sutures passed through the bone of the glenoid and around the labrum. This separation of the labrum from the glenoid is referred to as a Bankart lesion (Fig. 19.4), and the operation is referred to as a Bankart repair. In addition to this, the lax capsule of the front of the shoulder joint is tightened up by means of a double-breasting procedure referred to as the Putti–Platt procedure. Post-operatively the arm is immobilized in adduction and internal rotation for 6 weeks and then gradually progressive mobilization is begun. Recurrence of dislocation following this operation is rare.

RECOMMENDATIONS FOR FURTHER READING

BOYD, H. B. and HUNT, H. L. (1965) Recurrent dislocation of the shoulder, *J. Bone Jt Surg.* **47A**, 1514–20.

RANG, M. (1966) Original descriptions of methods of reducing shoulder dislocations, Hippocrates and Kocher. In *Anthology of Orthopaedics*, pp. 225–7, E. & S. Livingstone, Edinburgh.

RATHBUN, J. B. and MACNAB, I. (1970) The microvascular pattern of the rotator cuff, *J. Bone Jt Surg.* **52B**, 540–53.

20 The arm

There are two conditions for discussion which occur in the arm—spontaneous rupture of the tendon of biceps and fracture of the humerus.

SPONTANEOUS RUPTURE OF THE TENDON OF BICEPS

The biceps brachii muscle, as its name implies, has two heads, which take origin from two different parts of the scapula. The short head arises from the coracoid process and the long head from the upper surface of the glenoid fossa. The tendon of the long head of biceps passes through the capsule of the shoulder joint and down the bicipital groove on the anterior aspect of the upper humerus. As mentioned in Chapter 12, it occasionally becomes inflamed in this area and it is in this upper part of its tendon that it undergoes spontaneous rupture.

After the acute pain and swelling have settled, and they may be minimal, patient notices a difference in the shape of the front of his arm. This extra 'lump' is the released belly of the long head of biceps. It becomes more obvious if he contracts his biceps. This can be done by flexing the elbow against resistance or by supinating the forearm against resistance. The old name for the biceps was 'supinator longus'.

Treatment is not recommended as the loss of power is negligible. It is important to remember that the main flexor of the elbow is the brachialis muscle.

FRACTURES OF THE HUMERUS

Fractures of the humerus are common. They are due either to direct violence, e.g. in traffic accidents or to falls, in which case they are often caused by twisting strains and hence spiral in shape. They occur at all ages.

Treatment
Most fractures of the humerus are extremely mobile and the weight of the arm and forearm usually provides the traction necessary for reduction. Immobilization is by splintage. A long lateral splint is applied after being bent in such a way that it rests on the trapezius muscle at the base of the neck, then passes over the point of the shoulder and down the outer side of the arm to end about 2 cm below the point of the elbow. Two shorter straight splints are then applied to the antero-medial and the postero-medial aspects of the arm. All splints are applied over a generous thickness of splint wool and are held in position by strips of non-stretchable strapping. The elbow is held flexed to about 110° in a collar-and-cuff sling. Care must be taken to ensure that the

antero-medial splint does not cause undue pressure on the forearm flexor muscles.
This splintage must be checked weekly until the fracture has united.

Complications of fractures of the humerus

Damage to the radial nerve

The radial nerve winds round the shaft of the humerus in its middle third from the medial to the lateral side lying, as it does so, in the musculospiral groove (the old name for the radial nerve was the musculospiral nerve.) It is not surprising therefore that it is often damaged in fractures of the humerus.

Damage to the nerve at this level will lead to loss of dorsiflexion of the wrist ('wrist-drop'), loss of extension of the interphalangeal joint of the thumb, and loss of extension of the metacarpo-phalangeal joints of the fingers. The brachioradialis muscle will also be paralysed. This muscle is tested most easily by asking the patient to flex his elbow against resistance with the forearm in neutral rotation, i.e. thumb pointing upwards.

It is not unusual in oblique fractures of the humerus for the nerve to become displaced into the fracture line.

Treatment. The problem of treatment of radial paralysis in association with fractures of the humerus is one of deciding whether one is dealing with a complete division of the nerve (neurotmesis) or a lesion which will recover spontaneously (axonotmesis or neurapraxia). The general tendency is to adopt an expectant line of treatment checking for recovery in the brachioradialis muscle. If the fracture outline is such that one suspects entrapment of the nerve, exploration is indicated. Of course, if the fracture is compound the nerve may be easily identified. If one has adopted an expectant line of treatment and there has been no sign of nerve recovery at 3 months, exploration should be undertaken.

Sometimes it is found at operation that there has been extensive damage to the nerve and that continuity cannot be restored. In these cases the wound is closed and at a subsequent operation transplantation of wrist flexor tendons is carried out so that they act as thumb and finger extensors and extensors of the wrist.

Delayed union or non-union

Although it is rare, there is a definite incidence of non-union in fractures of the humerus. Some authorities believe that it exists because of the fact that effective immobilization of the proximal fragment is impossible.

The treatment of delayed union is by internal fixation and bone grafting. Internal fixation may be achieved by the use of a plate screwed on to the humeral shaft or by intermedullar nailing. There is, unfortunately, a small group of patients in whom even this method of treatment is unsuccessful and repeated operations may be necessray.

21 The elbow region

Anatomy

The elbow consists of two joints:
(1) a hinge joint between the humerus and the ulna;
(2) a shallow ball-and-socket joint between the capitellum and the head of the radius.

Although anatomically continuous with the elbow joint, the upper radio-ulnar joint is usually considered separately.

Important nomenclature

Figs 21.1, 21.2, and 21.3 show the names for the parts of the humerus, ulna, and radius. Note that the head of the radius is at its upper end but that the head of the ulna is at its lower end.

Ossification

The lower epiphysis of the humerus ossifies from four separate centres. A knowledge of the time of appearance of these secondary ossification centres for the lower humeral epiphysis and the upper epiphysis of the radius and ulna is important because these appear separate from the main bone on radiographs and are easily mistaken for fractures.

The centres for the lower end of the humerus appear in the following order:
1. Capitellum, appearing at about 3 years.
2. Internal epicondyle, appearing at about 5 years.
3. Trochlea, appearing at about 11 years.

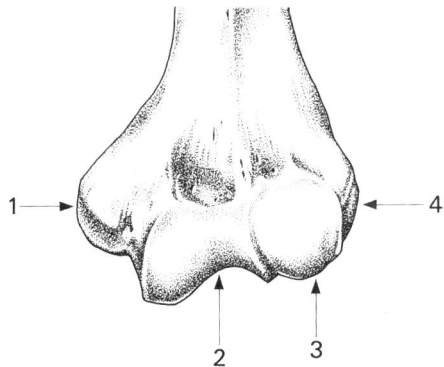

FIG. 21.1. The lower end of the humerus: (1) internal or medial epicondyle; (2) trochlea; (3) capitellum; (4) external or lateral epicondyle.

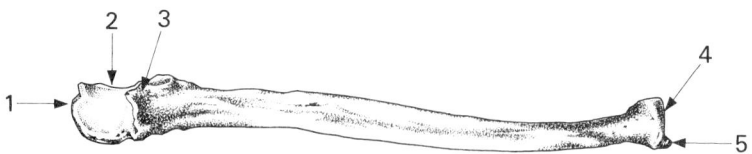

FIG. 21.2. Ulna: (1) olecranon process; (2) trochlear notch; (3) coronoid process; (4) head of ulna; (5) styloid process of ulna.

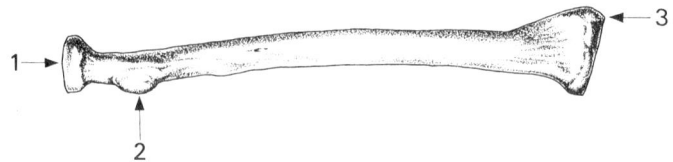

FIG. 21.3. Radius: (1) head of radius; (2) radial tubercle; (3) styloid process.

4. External epicondyle, appearing at about 13 years.

The centre for the upper ends of the radius appears at about 7 years and that for the upper end of the ulna (olecranon) at 9 years.

The time of appearance of these centres can be remembered by the mnemonic CIRUTE—the time of appearance being on alternate years from 3 to 13.

Movements

Flexion and extension of the elbow take place at the humero-ulnar and radio-capitellar joints. Pronation and supination at the radio-capitellar and upper and lower radio-ulnar joints.

Congenital radio-ulnar synostosis

In this condition there is a congenital bony bar across the upper radio-ulnar joint, preventing pronation and supination. Flexion and extension of the elbow are not affected. The loss of pronation can be compensated for by rotation at the shoulder. The loss of supination is the main disability. The condition tends to affect both elbows.

Treatment

Most children adapt well to any disability caused. Operative correction is usually unsuccessful because of associated soft-tissue defects.

Congenital dislocation of the radio-humeral joint

A rare condition resulting in some diminution in the range of flexion. Treatment is seldom needed and excision of the head of the radius, if considered necessary, should be postponed until growth of the skeleton is complete.

Arthro-gryposis multiplex congenita

The elbow is a common site for this condition. It is usually associated with other joint involvement, especially the knees, hips, and ankles.

Signs

The characteristic lack of skin creases and loss of muscle contour is seen. Joint movement is restricted.

Pathology
There is loss of differentiation of mesenchyme into muscle tendon and fascia.

Treatment
Periodic manipulation and splintage to prevent increase of the flexion deformity. In later life, soft-tissue release operations may be necessary to increase the range of movement or improve the position of the elbow.

DEFORMITIES OF THE ELBOW REGION

Cubitus valgus

An increase in the carrying angle may be congenital in origin but is more often due to mal-union of a supracondylar fracture of the humerus or to interference with the growth of part of the lower epiphyseal complex of the humerus—again following fractures. Progressive deformities, especially if severe, may cause traction on the ulnar nerve giving rise to paraesthesia, paresis, or paralysis in its area of distribution.

Cubitus varus

This deformity is less acceptable cosmetically than the valgus deformity and is usually caused by mal-union in supracondylar fractures of the humerus (Fig. 21.4).

Minor degrees of deformity do not require treatment. More severe types require osteotomy of the humerus.

Tuberculous arthritis of the elbow

This is rare now in Britain, but several cases of old infection which have gone on to bony ankylosis are still to be seen.

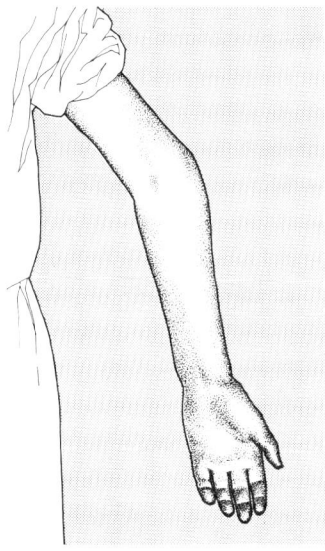

FIG. 21.4. Cubitus varus.

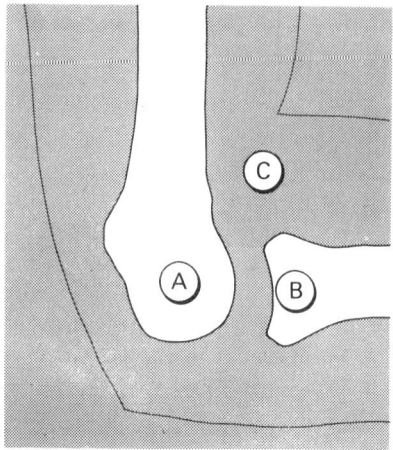

FIG. 21.5. Tennis elbow, showing common sites of tenderness.
A, the lateral humeral epicondyle.
B, the radio-humeral joint and head of radius.
C, the common extensor origin.

Tennis elbow

This is a very common condition which has a variety of causes.

Symptoms
The main symptom is pain which is felt over the outer side of the elbow and down the dorsal aspect of the forearm and hand. It is usually aggravated by use, e.g. shovelling coal or wringing washing.

Signs
There is tenderness over the lateral side of the elbow. This is maximal in one of three sites (Fig. 21.5):
   (1) the lateral epicondyle of the humerus (epicondylalgia);
   (2) the radio-humeral joint and the head of the radius;
   (3) the origin and upper bellies of the extensor muscles (brachio-radialis and extensor carpi radialis longus and brevis).

The finger extension test. The patient is asked to extend the fingers at the metacarpo-phalangeal joints against resistance. This may cause pain over the outer side of the elbow.

Mills' test. The examiner holds the patient's wrist flexed and then extends the elbow. Again, pain is felt over the outer side of the elbow.

Pathology
There are several causes of tennis elbow:
   (1) inflammation of the periosteum of the lateral humeral epicondyle or adjacent extensor muscle origin;
   (2) tears or sprains of the extensor muscle origin;
   (3) chrondromalacia of the radial head;
   (4) compression of the radial nerve as it passes over the lateral aspect of the elbow joint.

Treatment
Ultrasonic therapy is sometimes effective. Manipulation of the elbow with stretching of the extensors under general anaesthesia is often curative.

Injection of hydrocortisone into the tender area is probably the most effective method of treatment. If chondromalacia of the radial head is thought to be the cause, the injection should be given intra-articularly. In this case full aseptic technique should be used and the injection done in the operating theatre.

Severe tears of the extensor muscle origin may also involve the capsule of the elbow joint and require operative repair. Some authorities advise operative decompression of the radial nerve at the outer side of the elbow. The practice in our department consists of hydrocortisone injections, given peri-articularly or intra-articularly, dependiig on the side of the tenderness; up to a maximum of three injections. If symptoms persist after these injections, operative release of the common extensor origin is carried out.

Golfer's elbow

This term is used to describe a rarer condition similar to tennis elbow but occurring in the region of the medial epicondyle. The vast majority of cases respond to injection of hydrocortisone.

Olecranon bursitis (student's elbow)

An adventitious bursa may form over the upper end of the ulna where it is covered only by skin. This bursa may become distended with fluid or become inflamed.

Treatment
On the first occasion aspiration of the fluid may cause resolution of the condition. Surgical removal is indicated for recurrent effusions.

If infection supervenes it should be treated by aspiration and the administration of the appropriate antibiotic. Following resolution of the infection removal of the bursa is advised.

Osteochondritis dissecans

This condition occurs in the elbows of adolescents and young adults.

Symptoms
A vague discomfort or ache is felt in the elbow and, later, locking may occur due to the presence of a loose body. Flexion may also be limited.

Signs
Some resistance to movement or tenderness in the early stages. After the loose body has separated, synovial effusion, blocking the range of extension or flexion, are found and occasionally the loose body may be palpable.

Radiographs
These may show an irregular area in the articular surface of the trochlea, capitellum, or trochlear notch, or may demonstrate the loose body lying free in the joint.

Treatment

In the early stages, conservative treatment in the form of heat and mobilization exercises are beneficial. In the later stage the loose body or bodies may require removal.

Osteoarthrosis

This is seen in the elbow both in its secondary form (following injury or incongruity of joint surfaces) and, more rarely, in its primary form. The osteophytes formed may break off and come to lie loose in the joint. Effusions, sudden pain, and sudden loss of movement may occur.

Treatment

As the elbow is not a weight-bearing joint, pain relief can be obtained by resting, splintage, heat, and analgesics. With the exception of arthrodesis in exceptional cases, operative treatment of the condition is generally not required. However, loose bodies may require removal.

INJURIES IN THE ELBOW REGION

Fractures of the lateral humeral epicondyle

A small piece of bone may be fractured from the lateral part of the lower humerus. The fracture is often due to avulsion of the humeral attachment of the lateral ligament of the elbow caused by a varus strain. Usually it is not markedly displaced and treatment is by immobilization until union has occurred.

Fractures of the capitellum

These are more serious injuries and are seen commonly in children and young adults. Diagnosis may be difficult in the young because of the widely spaced centres of ossification. An added difficulty is that the fragment of bone or pre-bone cartilage becomes displaced and rotated and closed reduction is impossible (Fig. 21.6). Open reduction is therefore indicated and in adults the immobilization is achieved by inserting a small pin. In the young, the danger of interference with epiphyseal growth is minimized by using sutures through neighbouring soft tissues to achieve immobilization, rather than pin-fixation.

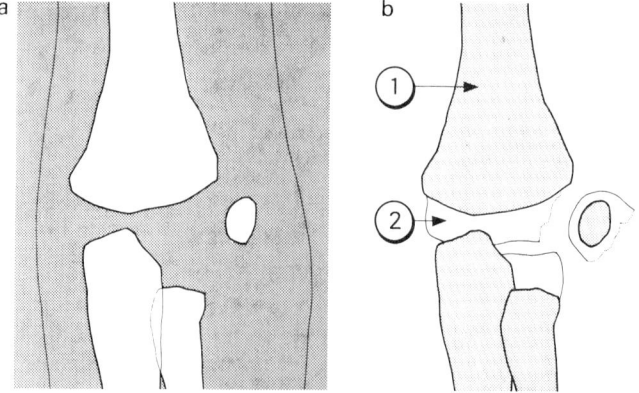

FIG. 21.6. Fracture of the capitellum in the child. (a) The radiographic appearance. (b) The actual injury: (1) bone; (2) pre-bone cartilage.

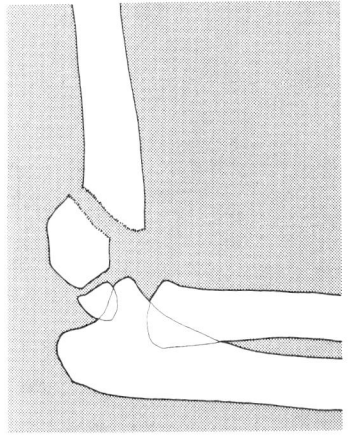

FIG. 21.7. Supracondylar fracture of the humerus.

Complications
1. A cubitus valgus deformity may result from mal-union or growth arrest.
2. Ulnar palsy may occur, either at the time of injury or later due to development of a valgus deformity.

Fractures of the medial humeral epicondyle
This lesion is similar to that seen in the lateral epicondyle and is due usually to avulsion of a small fragment of bone by a strain of the medial ligament of the elbow. Displacement is usually slight and no reduction is necessary.

Supracondylar fractures of the humerus
This fracture is commonly seen in children and causes grave concern to the orthopaedic surgeon because of the danger of damage to the brachial artery, with resultant ischaemia of the forearm and hand. The fracture is usually caused by a fall onto the outstretched hand. The fracture occurs in the lowest 2 or 3 cm of the humerus; the fracture line is horizontal but usually a spike of bone is found attached to the upper fragment at the medial or lateral end of the fracture line. The lower fragment is usually displaced posteriorly (Fig. 21.7).

Signs
Within the first few minutes of the injury the bony displacement may be palpable. However, soft-tissue swelling and oedema occur rapidly, causing difficulty both with diagnosis and management. There may be signs of a neurological deficit in the forearm—the median and the ulnar nerves being the most commonly involved. Ischaemia of the forearm is a serious complication (see p. 140).

Radiographs
These show the displacement described above. In the very young, the scarcity of ossified cartilage may make interpretation of the radiographic appearances difficult.

Treatment

The fracture can usually be reduced by manipulation. There is some debate as to whether the elbow joint should be held flexed or extended during manipulation, some authorities arguing that damage to the brachial artery is more likely if the elbow is held extended. The proponents of the 'extended-elbow school' argue that they have better control over the distal fragment and can apply more efficient traction with the limb held in this position.

After reduction, the triceps acts as an efficient splint, and it is necessary only to ensure that the elbow is flexed in order to achieve immobilization. This flexion is achieved by applying a collar-and-cuff sling. Some surgeons also protect the limb by means of a plaster of Paris backslab.

Occasionally open reduction of the fracture is necessary because of irreducibility due to the interposition of soft tissues between the fragments. Ischaemia of the forearm is discussed on p. 140.

Y-shaped and comminuted fractures of the lower humerus

These occur more frequently in adults than children and are usually caused by direct violence.

Treatment is by manipulative reduction and external fixation in a plaster of Paris cast. Occasionally, however, the degree of comminution makes accurate reduction impossible. In these cases, continuous gentle skeletal traction applied via a wire passed through the upper ulna usually results in an acceptable reduction and a remarkably wide range of subsequent elbow movement.

Fractures of the olecranon process of the ulna

In children and adolescents, a fracture separation of the olecranon epiphysis may occur. This may be due to direct violence or muscle pull by the triceps. If displaced, it should be reduced and held in position by sutures placed in the surrounding soft tissues, or through the bone well clear of the epiphyseal plate. Plaster of Paris fixation for 4–6 weeks is usually adequate.

In adults, the fracture line tends to be more distal and involve the trochlear notch. In these cases separation of the fragments is common. The olecranon fragment may be pulled up posterior to the humeral shaft by the triceps and the distal fragment (shaft of ulna) may be pulled up anterior to the humeral shaft by the biceps and brachialis (Fig. 21.8). The hinge action of the elbow joint will then be lost unless open reduction and fixation with an intramedullary screw are carried out.

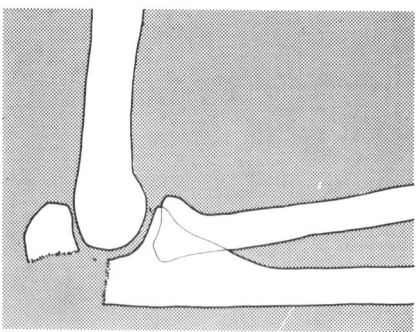

FIG. 21.8 Fracture of the olecranon.

Avulsion fractures of the coronoid process

These are rare and displacement is usually minimal. Treatment is by immobilization of the elbow until the pain has settled. Active movement is then encouraged.

Fractures of the neck of the radius

These occur following falls on the outstretched hand and are important as they may be angulated and, if allowed to unite in this position, may interfere with pronation and supination movements. Characteristically they occur in children and adolescents.

Manipulative reduction is usually successful but if not, open reduction may be indicated. Some degree of moulding may be expected in the less angulated fractures.

Fractures of the head of the radius

These fractures characteristically occur in adults. The usual cause is a fall on to the outstretched hand. The fractures may be single or comminuted. In the adult comminuted fractures are usually treated by excision of the radial head. Single fractures are often undisplaced and treated conservatively. Displaced small fragments may be excised.

In children, the radial head should not be excised until growth is complete because of the danger of the development of a valgus deformity of the elbow.

Dislocations of the elbow joint

This is a relatively common injury, seen in adults, and usually caused by falling onto the outstretched hand. The ulna is displaced posteriorly and either to the medial or the lateral side of the lower end of the humerus. The radiocapitellar joint is also dislocated. Nerve lesions are surprisingly rare.

Signs

The most dependable signs are the deformity, pain on attempted movement, and loss of the normal alignment of the olecranon process relative to the medial and lateral humeral epicondyles.

Treatment

Manipulative reduction under general anaesthesia is relatively simple and the joint is usually stable to all forces after reduction. Rest in a full-arm sling for 2–3 weeks is advisable.

Complication

A rare but serious complication is myositis ossificans—the presence of areas of ossification in the muscles surrounding the elbow. The cause is unknown but many surgeons attribute it to premature mobilization of the joint after injury.

The treatment recommended is rest until the pain which accompanies the appearance of these ossified areas has settled and then gentle exercise. Attempts to excise the new bone usually lead to further deposition of similar new bone.

Dislocation of the head of the radius

Although this lesion usually accompanies a fracture of the ulna (see

Monteggia fracture; p. 143) it occasionally occurs in isolation, especially in children.

Signs
On palpation of the outer side of the elbow the normal prominence of the radial head in front of the lateral humeral epicondyle cannot be felt and flexion of the elbow is deficient.

Radiographs
These confirm the diagnosis. In a lateral radiograph of the normal elbow, a line drawn along the centre of the shaft of the radius when extended upwards will pass through the centre of the capitellum. In a case of dislocation it passes through the humerus above the capitellum.

Treatment
In a case seen soon after injury, reduction is usually easy, but immobilization is difficult and redislocation or subluxation often occurs.

Operative repair of the annular ligament or replacement of it by a fascial sling may be necessary.

Volkmann's ischaemic contracture

Ischaemia of the forearm muscles may be seen in fractures and dislocations in the region of the elbow. It is commonest in supracondylar fractures of the humerus in children (p. 137).

The cause of the ischaemia is either actual division or occlusion of the brachial artery itself, or spasm caused by irritation or intimal damage to the vessel or others with which it communicates in the anastomosis around the elbow joint. This spasm may also be produced because of traction on a branch of the artery due to its being caught over the distal end of the proximal fragment.

The signs and symptoms of ischaemia may come on after reduction of the fracture.

Symptoms
Pain in the forearm and hand especially on moving the fingers.

Signs
These are as follows.
1. Loss of the wrist pulses (radial and ulnar).
2. Pallor of the hand and fingers.
3. Tenderness in the forearm on attempted straightening of the fingers. In a young child this can be elicited by stroking the flexor surface of the fingers.

Treatment
It is essential to re-establish circulation in the forearm and hand and this takes precedence over the treatment of the fracture.

1. The elbow should be gradually extended, watching for the return of the pulse at the wrist. Occasionally this necessitates complete extension of the elbow, and if this is necessary, immobilization of the fracture can be achieved by using a Thomas's arm splint.

Frequently this extension of the elbow is successful in re-establishing the circulation.

The elbow region   141

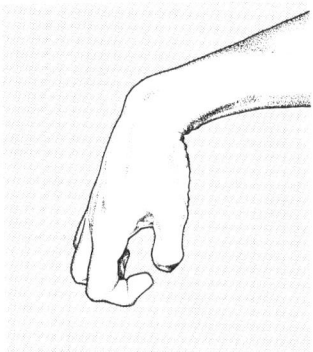

FIG. 21.9. The position of the hand
in Volkmann's ischaemic contracture.

2. If extension fails to re-establish the circulation, the artery should be explored. Surgical decompression and topical use of antispasmodic drugs (e.g. papaverine) is tried.
3. If, at operation, the circulation does not recover after decompression of the artery or release of its branches, resection of the damaged section of the artery usually leads to a dilatation of the other vessels in the anastomosis around the elbow joint with re-establishment of the circulation.
4. If the forearm flexor compartment is unduly tense, it should be decompressed by incision of its fascial sheath.

Late cases. The end result of untreated (or unsuccessfully treated) ischaemia is that the forearm muscles undergo necrosis and are replaced by fibrous tissue. Contraction of this fibrous tissue affects the forearm flexors more than the extensors, resulting in a characteristically deformed hand (Fig. 21.9). The metacarpo-phalangeal joints are extended, the interphalangeal joints flexed and the wrist usually partially flexed. The thumb is also held flexed. Forced passive flexion of the wrist may allow a small range of extension at the interphalangeal joints.

Treatment
The established case of Volkmann's contracture is treated by excision of the fibrosed areas and muscle-sliding operations to free the fingers and wrist. This results in improvement of hand function but the ultimate use of the hand is always somewhat restricted.

RECOMMENDATIONS FOR FURTHER READING

BOSWORTH, D. M. (1965) Surgical treatment of tennis elbow, *J. Bone Jt Surg.* **47A**, 1533–6.
RANG, M. (1966) Volkmann's ischaemic contracture, original description. In *Anthology of Orthopaedics*, pp. 88–90, E. & S. Livingstone, Edinburgh.
ROLES, N. C. and MAUDSLEY, R. H. (1972) Radial tunnel syndrome. Resistant tennis elbow as a nerve entrapment. *J. Bone Jt Surg.* **54B**, 499–508.
SHERWIN STAPLES, O. (1965) Dislocation of the brachial artery—A complication of supra-condylar fracture of the humerus in childhood, *J. Bone Jt Surg.* **47A**, 1525–32.

22 The forearm

ANATOMY

The most important function of the forearm is that of pronation and supination. In its simplest form this is a movement of the radius around the ulna, the ulna being the axis of rotation. You can demonstrate this simple action by laying the forearm on a table and rotating it from full pronation to full supination. It will be noted that the axis of rotation is the line of the ulna or little finger.

In everyday use of forearm pronation and supination the axis of rotation is not the line of the little finger but usually the line of the thumb or index finger. This means that some slight extension and flexion movement takes place at the elbow joint and some lateral and medial rotation movement at the shoulder joint. The main movements, however, still take place at the upper and lower radio-ulnar joints. For proper movements after trauma, therefore, we need functional radio-ulnar joints and a radius and ulna that can be rotated about each other over a range of 180°.

RADIAL CLUB HAND

Some children are born without a radius in one or either forearm. In some it may be partially present and in others the thumb ray is also absent (Fig. 22.1). With growth of the ulna the hand becomes angulated towards the radial side hence the name 'radial club hand'. In some of these children the elbow joint is also deformed and may be stiff. The ulna is usually shorter than normal.

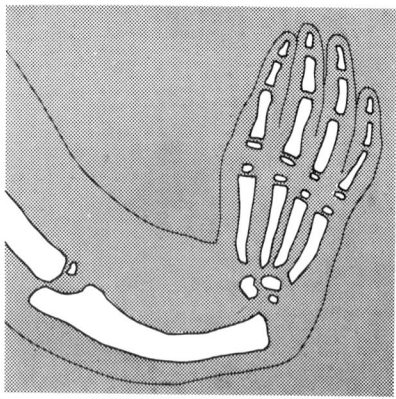

FIG. 22.1. The radiographic appearance of radial club hand.

Treatment

The aim of treatment is to obtain the maximum functional ability of the forearm and hand.

If the elbow is stiff most surgeons would advise against straightening the hand on the forearm because this would probably prevent the child from getting his hand to his mouth. If there is a good range of elbow movement, early stretching and splintage is employed to keep the deformity to a minimum. Later, the appearance and function of the hand may be improved by soft-tissue release on the radial side (there is often a fibrous band replacing the radius) followed by centralization of the carpus on the ulna and fusing it in this position.

However, the child may opt not to have the operation as many of them are remarkably dextrous with their radial club hands.

FRACTURES OF THE FOREARM BONES

Isolated fractures

Isolated fractures of the radius and the ulna do occur, especially due to direct injury. If the radio-ulnar joint alignment has not been upset and reduction to a position of no abnormal angulation can be achieved, manipulative reduction and external fixation (splints or plaster cast) is satisfactory. It is important to note that some displacement is acceptable as it does not subsequently interfere with pronation and supination, but angulation is usually not acceptable because it does interfere with rotation.

Greenstick fracture of radius and ulna

This fracture is seen very commonly in paediatric practice. The fact that one cortex of the bone is intact means that displacement is not a problem although angulation may be. Most of these fractures can be gently manipulated back into position without much difficulty. External fixation is adequate. It must be emphasized that all fractures of the forearm bones, with the exception of those in the lowest inch of the bones, should be immobilized in splints or plaster casts which extend from the axilla to the metacarpal heads and hold the elbow at a right-angle.

Fractures of both bones of the forearm

Complete fractures occur both in children and in adults. They are remarkably difficult to reduce and even more difficult to hold. Although we try to treat these fractures by manipulative reduction and external fixation we quite often have to resort to open reduction and/or internal fixation. Plates or Rush intermedullary nails are the common methods used. It should be pointed out that with closed reduction and external fixation a very close follow-up is required, the patient being seen and the fracture X-rayed every week for 4–5 weeks.

Monteggia fracture

This name is given to a combination of injuries: a fracture of the ulna, usually in its upper third, associated with dislocation of the superior radio-ulnar joint (Fig. 22.2). Two types are described: in the first the distal fragment of

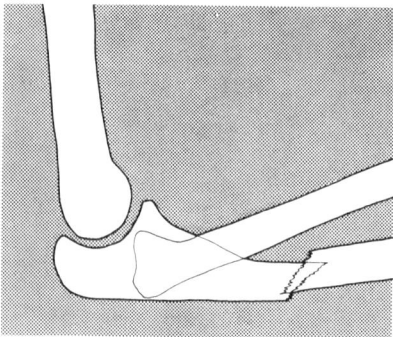

FIG. 22.2. Monteggia fracture.

the ulna is angulated forwards and the head of the radius dislocated posteriorly (Monteggia in flexion). In the second the distal fragment of the ulna is angulated backwards and the head of the radius is dislocated forwards (Monteggia in extension). Both are, in fact, due to rotation injuries of the forearm.

Treatment

Reduction of the ulnar fracture usually results in reduction of the upper radio-ulnar joint. In some adults open reduction of the radio-ulnar joint and repair of the annular ligament may be necessary. Most Monteggia fractures can be held with external fixation but instability to compression or angulation indicates that internal fixation is advisable.

Galeazzi fracture

This fracture is the opposite of the Monteggia fracture, namely a fracture of the radius with dislocation of the lower radio-ulnar joint (Fig. 22.3). Reduction of the radial fracture results in reduction of the lower radio-ulnar joint. It should be remembered that the articular surface of the lower end of the radius is about an eighth of an inch distal to the lower end of the ulna, so that if the radiograph shows them at the same level the lower radio-ulnar joint is displaced.

The fracture line of the radial fracture is often oblique and the fracture therefore unstable to compression. In these cases external fixation is unlikely to hold the fracture and internal fixation (plate or Rush pin) is indicated.

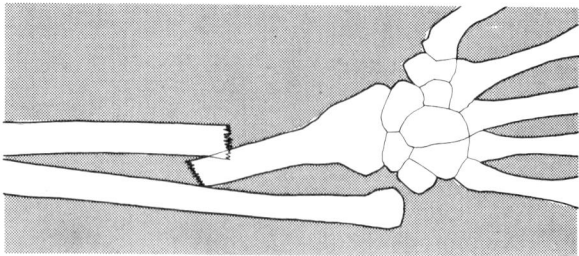

FIG. 22.3. Galeazzi fracture.

Fracture of the lower third of the radius and ulna in children
This is one of the more difficult childhood fractures to reduce and hold. It is sometimes referred to as the pronator fracture as it occurs at the level of attachment of pronator quadratus. Reduction may be difficult and the distal fragment may show a tendency to angulate dorsally after reduction. This may be prevented by immobilization in full arm splints or a plaster cast with the elbow flexed to 90° and the forearm in full supination.

It has been traditional in our practice to immobilize forearm fractures in full supination if consistent with maintaining reduction. The philosophy is that if rotation is lost it is better to have the forearm in some degree of supination because pronation can be replaced by shoulder abduction and internal rotation. Compensatory movement at the shoulder does not exist for a forearm stiff in pronation.

RECOMMENDATIONS FOR FURTHER READING

RANG, M. (1966) Monteggia and Galeazzi fractures, original description. In *Anthology of Orthopaedics*, p. 97, E. & S. Livingstone, Edinburgh.

23 The wrist region

ANATOMY

The wrist joint is the joint between the lower end of the radius and the proximal row of carpal bones. The lower end of ulna does not take part in the wrist joint directly as it is covered by the triangular cartilage.

Other joints are present in the wrist region:
(1) the transverse carpal joint between the proximal and distal rows of the carpal bones;
(2) the lower radio-ulnar joint;
(3) the carpo-metacarpal joints, of which the most important from the orthopaedic point of view is that of the thumb—between the trapezium and the base of the thumb metacarpal.

The movements of the wrist joint are dorsiflexion, palmar flexion, and ulnar and radial deviation. The lower radio-ulnar joint takes part (with the upper) in the movements of pronation and supination. Some dorsiflexion and palmarflexion movement occurs at the transverse carpal joint and this range is often increased in patients whose wrist joints have become ankylosed (stiffened by natural processes) or have been arthrodesed (stiffened operatively).

The carpal bones

Students often find difficulty in remembering the names of the bones of the carpus. Look at your own right palm or the skeleton of a hand, and start at the left end of the distal row of carpal bones. The names of the bones as one moves in a clockwise direction are shown in Fig. 23.1. This can be remembered by the mnemonic 'Hamlet came to town shouting loudly to Polonius'.

The thumb metacarpal articulates with the trapezium and the lower end of the radius articulates mainly with the scaphoid. From the clinical point of view, the important bones are the trapezium (osteoarthrosis), the scaphoid (fractures), and the lunate (dislocations and Keinbock's disease).

CLINICAL CONDITIONS IN THE WRIST REGION

Madelung's deformity

Madelung in 1879 described a condition in which the normal growth pattern of the lower end of the radius is upset by premature fusion of the medial part of the lower radial epiphysis. With the growth of the child, the radius becomes progressively bowed and at completion of growth shows a posterior bowing and the lower end is also curved towards the ulna. This makes the lower end of the ulna more prominent. Inhibition of growth of the medial part of the lower radial epiphysis also means that the carpus comes to lie in a V-shaped

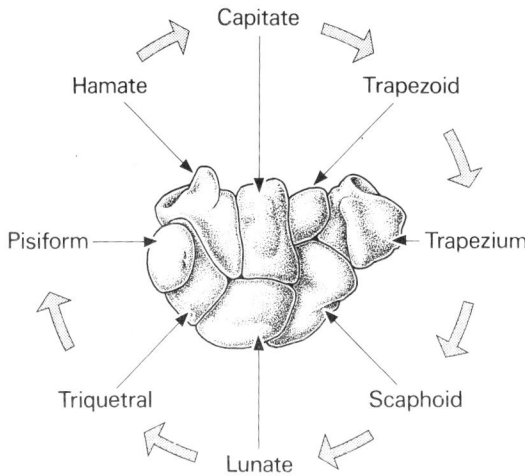

FIG. 23.1. The carpal bones.

notch formed by the lower ends of the radius and ulna. Flexion of the wrist is increased but other movements are restricted.

In modern usage the name Madelung has become associated with the deformity of undue prominence of the head of the ulna from any cause. Epiphyseal plate damage due to trauma or infection in the young and fractures of the lower end of the radius at any age may lead to the condition.

Shortening of the ulna or excision of its lower end are the methods of treatment in common use today.

De Quervain's syndrome

This condition is characterized by pain, swelling, and tenderness of the region of the radial styloid. The pain can be brought on by forced flexion of the thumb and it often radiates down the dorsal aspect of the thumb. It is common in middle-aged women and is due to a chronic tenosynovitis of the sheaths of the tendons of extensor pollicis brevis and abductor pollicis longus. Treatment is by excision of part of the thickened sheath to allow free movement of the tendons.

Mild cases may respond satisfactorily to an injection of hydrocortisone.

Subacute tenosynovitis

Painful swelling on the dorsum of the wrist and hand is sometimes encountered in people who find they have suddenly to use their hands more than they are used to doing. It is seen quite commonly in girls who take up nursing during their first months of training.

Examination reveals tenderness in these areas and crepitus on moving the fingers. The underlying condition is inflammation of the tendon sheaths on the dorsum of the hand and wrist.

Immobilization of the wrist and fingers on a splint usually cures the condition.

Ganglia

As mentioned in Chapter 12, ganglia are likely to occur on the dorsum of the wrist, indeed, this is the commonest site for their appearance. They are common in young women and their appearance may be preceded by vague aching at this site. Excision is advised, but there is a definite danger of recurrence.

Another common site for ganglia to occur is on the ventral aspect of the wrist deep to the radial artery. Delicate dissection during excision is needed in order to avoid damage to the artery.

The carpal tunnel syndrome

This is described in Chapter 5 (p. 30).

Keinbock's disease

This name is given to the condition of osteochondritis of the lunate. It is a disease of young men. The symptoms caused are aching and stiffness. Progression to osteoarthrosis of the wrist may occur. Symptomatic treatment is given in the early stages, but later the degenerative arthrosis may require treatment. In severe cases arthrodoesis may be necessary.

Septic arthritis

This is a relatively rare condition, seen mainly in children in association with osteomyelitis of the lower radius or carpus.

Tuberculous arthritis

The wrist was one of the commoner joints to be affected by tuberculosis and cases are still occasionally seen. Untreated, the condition leads to complete destruction of the carpal bones with abscess and sinus formation and fibrous ankylosis of the wrist. Treatment, if started early, may lead to a complete cure.

Rheumatoid disease

The wrist joints rank second only to the small joints of the fingers in frequency of affection.

Clinical signs

The synovium is usually thickened and the swelling is palpable on both the dorsal and the ventral surfaces. It is sometimes difficult to decide how much of the swelling on the dorsum of the wrist is due to swelling of the wrist joint synovium and how much is due to involvement of the tendon sheaths of the finger and wrist extensor tendons.

Spontaneous rupture of tendons is common and usually starts with the extensors of the little finger and later involves those of the ring, middle, and index fingers.

In the more acute stages wrist movement is painful and secondary degenerative arthritis is common in the later stages.

Radiographs

These show generalized loss of bone density and, later, localized areas of erosion—usually near articular surfaces and classically in the ulnar styloid. The signs of degenerative arthritis may supervene.

Treatment
Synovectomy often gives very satisfactory results and, as far as the extensor tendons are concerned, may prevent spontaneous rupture. The general treatment of rheumatoid disease was discussed in Chapter 6.

Degenerative arthrosis
Primary osteoarthrosis is uncommon in the wrist joint but common in the carpo-metacarpal joint of the thumb. The explanation for this is unknown but the suggestion has been made that it is because this joint is in constant use throughout the full range of its movement: this leads to repeated minor strains of the joint and hence to osteoarthrosis.

Symptoms
The patient complains of pain at the base of the thumb on using it and of a restriction in the range of extension and abduction. This may be a severe disability in manual workers and piano-players.

Treatment
Conservative treatment with heat, exercises, and intra-articular injections of hydrocortisone often relieve the pain. Intractable pain and stiffness may warrant removal of the trapezium.

Secondary osteoarthrosis is common in the wrist joint and is seen following rheumatoid arthritis and trauma—particularly fractures involving the articular surfaces of the lower end of the radius and the scaphoid.

INJURIES OF THE WRIST

Ligament and capsule sprains
These are particularly common in sports injuries and usually respond to rest and support with strapping. The diagnosis of a sprain should always be viewed with suspicion if the patient has fallen on to the outstretched hand and care should be taken to exclude a fracture of the scaphoid.

Fracture-separations of the lower radial epiphysis
These injuries, seen in children, are caused by falls on the outstretched hand. The wrist assumes the dinner-fork deformity, and radiographs show the displaced epiphysis and usually the triangular metaphyseal fragment which is carried with the epiphysis. Reduction follows the same manoeuvres as are used for the Colles' fracture and union usually occurs after 3–4 weeks of immobilization in splints.

Colles' fractures
These are the commonest fractures seen in modern orthopaedic practice. They occur in adults and are again caused by falls on the outstretched hand. The radius is fractured within an inch of its lower articular surface, and the ulna styloid process is usually fractured as well. The distal radial fragment is displaced dorsally and angulated dorsally and to the radial side (Fig. 23.2). This results in the characteristically 'humped' appearance of the wrist usually referred to as a 'dinner-fork deformity' (Fig. 23.3).

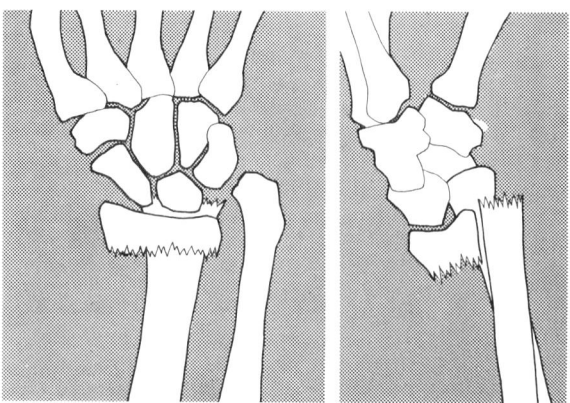

FIG. 23.2. Displaced Colles' fracture.

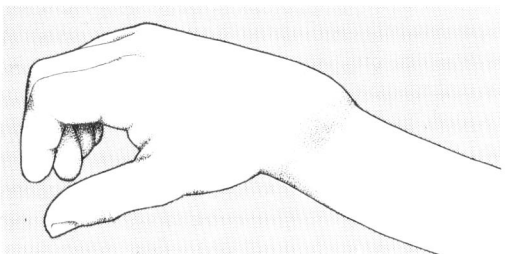

FIG. 23.3. Colles' fracture, showing the characteristic 'dinner-fork' deformity.

Treatment

Reduction is carried out under general anaesthesia. Traction is applied to the limb to disimpact the fracture. The distal fragment of the radius is then manipulated forward and to the ulnar side. Immobilization is achieved either by the use of a plaster backslab which is later converted to a forearm cast when the swelling has subsided, or by the use of a dorsal and a ventral splint which are applied over splint wool and held in position with non-stretch strapping. The use of splints is recommended provided the clinic staff understand the principles of their use. Frequent checks are needed to ensure that the splints are sufficiently tight and that finger movement is being practised. It is important also in all forearm fractures whether treated in splints or plaster casts to ensure that the patient retains a full range of shoulder movement by encouraging him or her to move the shoulder through its full range at least 3 times a day.

Smith's fractures

These, like the Colles' fractures, are confined to the lower inch of the radius but in Smith's fractures the displacement and angulation of the distal fragment is towards the ventral or palmar aspect of the wrist (Fig. 23.4).

Treatment

Reduction is again achieved by manipulation after preliminary traction to

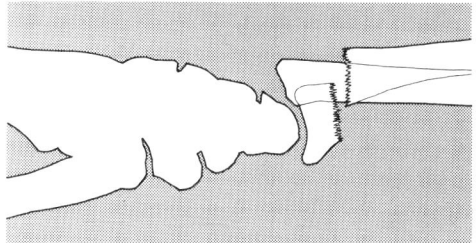

FIG. 23.4. Smith's fracture.

disimpact the fracture but immobilization is more difficult than in the case of the Colles' fracture and a full arm plaster-cast in full supination or full arm splintage in full supination is necessary. The latter is achieved by using a ventral splint which has a right-angle bend in it to fit the ventral aspects of the arm and forearm and a straight dorsal forearm splint. Periodic splint checks are necessary.

Barton's fractures

These again are fractures of the lower end of the radius and are considered by some authorities to be a type of Smith's fracture. The difference, however, is that the fracture line involves the articular surface of the lower end of the radius, usually in the coronal plane, i.e. across its wider diameter (Fig. 23.5). The dorsal cortex of the lower end of the radius remains intact and the ventral fragment displaces in a palmar direction. The carpus moves with the small ventral fragment.

Treatment

The displacement is usually relatively easy to reduce by manipulation but it may be impossible to maintain the reduction by external means. It is our practice to use a T-shaped buttress plate, named after Ellis of Southampton, to hold these fractures in the reduced position. The vertical stem of the T has two holes for screws which fix it to the shaft of the radius while the solid cross

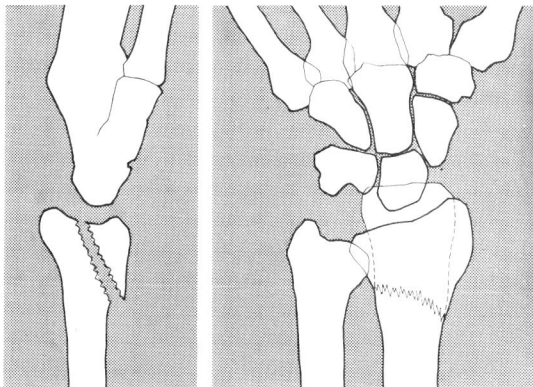

FIG. 23.5. Barton's fracture.

piece of the T holds the distal fragment in position against the intact dorsal cortex of the radius. Plaster fixation is used in addition to immobilize the wrist and elbow until the fracture has united.

Fractures of the styloid process of the radius

The radial styloid process may be fractured in injuries resulting from an acute radial deviation strain. The vast majority are minimally displaced and therefore can be treated by immobilization using splints or plaster. Very occasionally a large displaced fragment may require open reduction and screw fixation.

Fractures of the scaphoid bone

Fractures of the scaphoid bone are unique for two reasons:
(1) radiographs taken at the time of the injury may be deceptive;
(2) the unusual blood-supply may lead to avascular necrosis of the proximal fragment.

These fractures are common in young adult men and are usually caused by falls on to the outstretched hand. They are therefore common in Rugby football players. Fisk has shown that the fracture line in the scaphoid bone constitutes part of the line of disruption of the carpus as a whole.

Clinical features

Initial examination may reveal some swelling of the wrist, but there is no obvious alteration in its shape. There is usually tenderness over the dorsum of the wrist and characteristically in the floor of the 'anatomical snuff box'. Extension of the interphalangeal joint of the thumb may be deficient as pointed out by Stanley. Movements of the wrist are painful.

Radiographs

The fracture line across the waist of the scaphoid bone may be visible in one of the three views routinely taken: antero-posterior; lateral; and oblique (Fig. 23.6). Sometimes, however, there is no evidence of a fracture line. This is because of the nature of the scaphoid bone, which has a very thin cortex and a cancellous medulla.

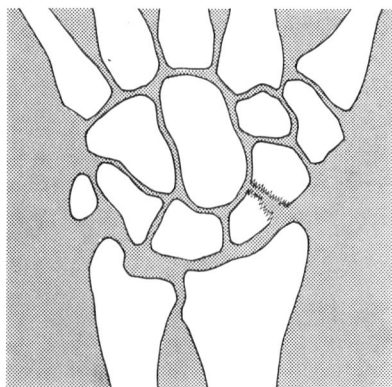

FIG. 23.6. Displaced fracture of the scaphoid bone.

Treatment

Fractures of the scaphoid bone are treated in forearm plaster casts which differ from the Colles' fracture casts in that the thumb is included. It is important that the terminal phalanx should be included in the cast. If the cast ends at the interphalangeal joint, the patient may 'hitch' the terminal phalanx of his thumb over the edge of the plaster and then, by flexing and extending the interphalangeal joint, produce traction on the thumb. This traction is transferred along the metacarpal to the trapezium and thence to the distal fragment of the scaphoid bone causing distraction of the fracture line with the consequent danger of delayed union.

If the clinical findings suggest a fracture of the scaphoid bone but the radiograph does not demonstrate it, it is wise to treat the wrist as though there was a fracture. It is immobilized in a scaphoid cast for 2 weeks. The cast is then removed and further radiographs taken. If the scaphoid bone is the site of a fracture, the radiograph taken at 2 weeks will almost certainly demonstrate it. The osteoporosis of early fracture healing will make it more obvious. If the 2-week film does not show a fracture it is usually safe to allow the patient to mobilize the wrist and then to use it normally.

Fractures of the scaphoid bone should be immobilized for at least 6 weeks and may well take up to 9–12 weeks to unite. The radiological assessment of union may be difficult.

Complications

Avascular negrosis of the proximal fragment. The arterial supply of the scaphoid arises from the radial artery and passes into the distal part of the scaphoid bone and thence to the proximal part. Damage to the artery in fractures across the waist of the scaphoid bone results therefore in avascular necrosis of the proximal part of the bone. This will, in time, cause irregularity of the articulation between the carpus and the lower end of the radius with consequent degenerative arthrosis. For this reason excision of the proximal pole is advised by some authorities. Grafting of the fracture may lead to revascularization. Established osteoarthrosis of this joint may be treated by excision of the styloid process of the radius.

Delayed union of fractures of the scaphoid bone. This may be due to ischaemia or inadequate immobilization. Treatment is by the insertion of a bone graft.

The grafts are usually taken from the lower radius or the subcutaneous border of the upper ulna.

It is important to realize that the discussion above refers to fractures of the waist of the scaphoid bone. Isolated fractures of the tuberosity, for example, are not affected by considerations of blood-supply and usually unite satisfactorily.

Fractures of the lunate bone

These are relatively rare injuries. They result from acute dorsiflexion strains of the wrist. There is swelling and tenderness over the dorsal aspect of the wrist.

The radiographic findings are characteristic. In the lateral view a small flake of bone can be seen on the dorsal aspect of the carpus.

Treatment by simple immobilization either in splints or in a forearm plaster cast is usually successful.

Dislocations of the wrist

Pure dislocations of the wrist are exceedingly rare. The usual series of events is that the carpus is disrupted in such a way that the lunate bone remains in normal relationship with the radius while the rest of the carpus is dislocated dorsally. The carpus then returns to its normal position and in doing so pushes the lunate forwards and tips it through 90°. This causes the characteristic change in the shape of the lunate as seen on the antero-posterior radiograph: it becomes triangular instead of moon-shaped. The injury is referred to as a 'perilunate dislocation of the wrist'. Closed manipulation and immobilization of the wrist in flexion may be successful but open reduction is often necessary.

Sometimes the line of disruption of the carpus instead of passing round the lunate bone passes through the waist of the scaphoid bone in addition to passing around the medial and distal aspects of the lunate bone. The resulting injury is referred to as a 'trans-scaphoid perilunate dislocation of the wrist'.

The principles of treatment are similar to those used for a perilunate dislocation but the added problems of the scaphoid fracture reduce the prospects of a successful outcome of treatment.

RECOMMENDATIONS FOR FURTHER READING

ELLIS, J. (1965) Smith's and Barton's fractures, *J. Bone Jt Surg.* **47B**, 724–7.

FISK, G. R. (1970) Carpal instability and the fractured scaphoid, *Ann. R. Coll. Surg.* **46**, 63–76.

RANG, M. (1966) Madelung's deformity, original description. In *Anthology of Orthopaedics*, pp. 36–8, E. & S. Livingstone, Edinburgh.

RANG, M. (1966) Colles' and Smith's fractures, original description. In *Anthology of Orthopaedics*, pp. 90–3, E. & S. Livingstone, Edinburgh.

24 The hand and fingers

ANATOMY

A knowledge of the action of the various muscles which act on the fingers and thumb and their nerve supply is essential for the understanding of the effects of peripheral nerve injuries on the hand.

The fingers

The joints involved in finger movement are:
  (1) the joint between the metacarpal and the proximal phalanx—the metacarpo-phalangeal (or m.p.) joint;
  (2) the joint between the proximal phalanx and the middle phalanx—the proximal interphalangeal (or p.i.p.) joint;
  (3) the joint between the middle phalanx and the distal phalanx—the distal interphalangeal (or d.i.p.) joint, sometimes referred to as the terminal interphalangeal (or t.i.p.) joint.

The movements of adduction and abduction of the fingers take place at the metacarpo-phalangeal joints. Adduction and abduction occur with reference to the middle finger, adduction being movement towards it and abduction being movement away from it.

Flexion and extension take place at all three joints—the metacarpo-phalangeal, the proximal interphalangeal, and the distal interphalangeal.

The thumb

The thumb differs from the other digits in three respects.

  1. Its position at rest is one of $90°$ of medial rotation as compared with the other digits. This becomes obvious if one notices the directions in which the nails are facing.
  2. It has only two phalanges and therefore only one interphalangeal joint.
  3. The joint between the metacarpal and the carpus (the carpo-metacarpal or trapezio-metacarpal joint) is much more mobile than those of the fingers. Abduction and adduction occur here, in a plane at right-angles to that of the abduction and adduction of the fingers, and in addition a certain amount of rotation is also possible at this joint. This is necessary for the function of opposition or the placing together of the pulps of finger and thumb. The actual movements of the thumb taking place in opposition are:
      (a) flexion (at carpo-metacarpal, metacarpo-phalangeal, and interphalangeal joints);
      (b) slight abduction (at the carpo-metacarpal joint);
      (c) medial rotation (at the carpo-metacarpal joint).

Muscles

Finger muscles

1. The metacarpo-phalangeal joints are flexed by the interossei and lumbricals acting together. The interossei arise between the metacarpals and insert into the bases of the proximal phalanges. There are three palmar and four dorsal interossei. The palmar interossei adduct the fingers and the dorsal interossei abduct the fingers.

The lumbricals arise from the tendons of flexor digitorum profundus as they traverse the palm and insert into the extensor espansions of the fingers. They pass on the radial side of the respective m.p. joints.

The metacarpo-phalangeal joints are extended by the extensor digitorum longus (old name: extensor digitorum communis).

2. The proximal interphalangeal joints are flexed by the flexor digitorum superficialis (old name: flexor digitorum sublimis).

The proximal interphalangeal joints are extended by the lumbricals and interossei which are referred to together as the small or intrinsic muscles of the hand.

3. The distal interphalangeal joints are flexed by the flexor digitorum profundus and extended by the lumbricals and interossei (small or intrinsic muscles of the hand).

Thumb-joint muscles

1. The metacarpo-phalangeal joint is flexed by flexor pollicis brevis and extended by extensor pollicis brevis.

2. The interphalangeal joint is flexed by flexor pollicis longus and extended by extensor pollicis longus.

3. The complex movements of the carpo-metacarpal joint are carried out by abductor pollicis longus, adductor pollicis, and the opponens pollicis.

Intrinsic muscles

It will be noted from the description of muscles acting on the fingers that the same group of muscles (lumbricals and interossei) produce two actions: they flex the m.p. joints and extend the i.p. joints. If acting normally these muscles produce flexion to 90° at the m.p. joints and extension at the i.p. joints. This is referred to as the 'intrinsic plus' position and this term implies normal function of these muscles. It is also the position in which babies are taught to wave goodbye and therefore unofficially called the 'ta-ta' position; The lumbricals and interossei which produce this position have the unofficial title of 'ta-ta' muscles (Fig. 24.1).

Paralysis of these muscles leads to the hand's adopting the opposite position of hyperextension of the m.p. joints (due to unopposed action of the extensor digitorum longus) and flexion of the p.i.p. and d.i.p. joints (due to unopposed action of flexor digitorum profundus and superficialis).

With the fingers in this position, the hand is referred to as the 'intrinsic minus' hand. It is also referred to as a 'claw hand'.

Motor nerve supply

The flexor digitorum superficialis is supplied by the median nerve. The flexor digitorum profundus has a double nerve supply: the part of the muscle moving the ring and little fingers is supplied by the ulnar nerve and the part moving the index and middle fingers by the median nerve.

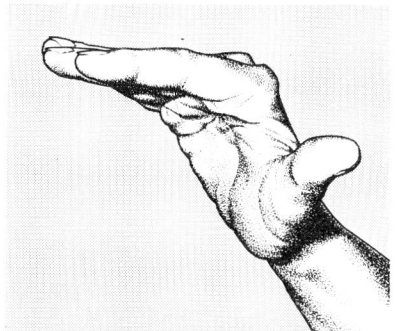

FIG. 24.1 The 'intrinsic plus' or 'ta-ta' position of the fingers.

The lumbricals are supplied by the same nerve as supplies the muscle bellies activating the tendons from which they arise: the little and ring finger lumbricals being supplied by the ulnar nerve and the index and middle finger lumbricals being supplied by the median nerve. The interossei are supplied by the ulnar nerve. The muscles of the thenar eminence are supplied by the median nerve through its recurrent branch.

The flexor pollicis longus is supplied by the median nerve and extensor pollicis longus and abductor pollicis longus by the radial nerve via its posterior interosseous branch.

From the above it will be obvious why damage to the ulnar nerve will lead to clawing (or the intrinsic minus position) of the ring and little finger.

Sensory nerve supply

Unfortunately the sensory supply of the hand and fingers does not correspond to the motor supply.

On the palmar aspect, the thumb, the radial half of the palm, the index finger, the middle finger, and the radial half of the ring finger are supplied by the median nerve. The area of supply extends onto the dorsal aspects of the fingers. The ulnar half of the ring finger both palmar and dorsal aspects, the palmar and dorsal aspects of the ulnar side of the hand, and the whole of the little finger are supplied by the ulnar nerve. A small part of the dorsum of the hand is supplied by the radial nerve.

CLINICAL CONDITIONS OF THE HAND AND FINGERS

Syndactyly

This is a congenital condition in which separation of the fingers is partially or totally deficient. It usually affects two fingers and radiographs usually show normally formed phalanges. The treatment is surgical separation of the conjoined fingers with various procedures including advancements and free skin grafts to cover the denuded areas of the fingers.

Congenital contracture of the little finger

The contracture usually affects the proximal interphalangeal joint which lacks about 30° of extension. It may be bilateral. It is important to distinguish this condition from Dupuytren's contracture because surgical treatment is not indicated in congenital contracture and results are disappointing, whereas Dupuytren's contracture can be cured by excision of the thickened palmar fascia. In the congenital contracture, the metacarpo-phalangeal joint is often held in a position of hyperextension.

Dupuytren's contracture

This condition was first described by Dupuytren, a French surgeon practising in Paris in the first half of the nineteenth century. It is a thickening and contracture of the palmar aponeurosis. The aponeurosis extends as a fan-shaped structure from the flexor retinaculum at the wrist to the level of the metacarpophalangeal joints and then sends slips into the fingers to attach to the middle phalanges. It also sends slips deeply to attach to the metacarpals themselves (Fig. 24.2).

The contracture starts as a small nodule usually opposite the base of the ring finger. It occasionally remains localized to this site. More commonly, however, it extends into the fingers and back towards the wrist presenting as a cord-like band. Adhesion to the skin is also common. With the passage of time, the band contracts and causes a flexion contracture first of the proximal interphalangeal joint and later of the metacarpo-phalangeal joint. The distal interphalangeal joint is not affected.

The contractures are sometimes so severe that the finger is permanently fixed in the palm. Although the ring finger is the commonest to be affected, any or all of the fingers may be affected. It is not unusual for the ring and little finger to be affected together.

Prognosis

As with most hand surgery, the most difficult joint to deal with is the proximal interphalangeal joint. If this joint has been held in a position of 90° or more of flexion for more than a few months it is highly unlikely that we will be able to restore its extension.

The opposite can be said of the metacarpo-phalangeal joint. This joint can

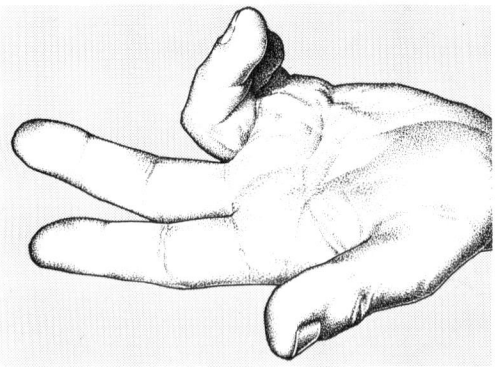

FIG. 24.2. Dupuytren's contracture affecting the ring and little finger.

be immobilized in a position of 90° flexion for many months and when the immobilizing agent is removed a full range of extension is regained.

The difference in the two joints lies in their collateral capsular ligaments. Those of the metacarpo-phalangeal joint are tight when the joint is flexed but loose when it is extended. This can be easily checked on your own fingers by measuring the degree of abduction and adduction possible with the joint in the two positions—extended and flexed to 90°. When the joint is immobilized for a long time, some contraction of the capsule occurs. If the joint on being released moves into a position where the capsule and ligaments are looser (extension in this case), none of the range of movement is lost.

In the p.i.p. joint the ligaments are tight in all positions of the joint so that it tends to stiffen in the position in which it is immobilized, hence extension is not regained if it has been fixed in flexion for a length of time.

Treatment
In early cases (before p.i.p. flexion contracture reaches 60–70°), good results can be expected from operative treatment. The operation aims at removing all the affected fascia, i.e. it is a fasciectomy.

It is normally done through a longitudinal incision which has cross-cuts made across it in order that it can be sutured as a multiple Z-plasty incision and so avoid difficulties due to shortage of skin or scar contracture. Care must be taken to avoid damage to the digital nerves which may be intimately involved with the thickened fascia. Early post-operative movement is recommended.

If the skin has been widely involved it may not be viable when dissected free from the 'Dupuytren tissue'. If this occurs over the palm there is seldom any serious consequence and new skin grows in quickly. If it occurs over the proximal phalanx, however, resulting fibrosis may cause recurrence of the contracture of the p.i.p. joint. In these cases excision of doubtful areas of skin and replacement with a full thickness skin graft is advisable.

Fasciotomy. In the past the operation of 'fasciotomy' was popular. In this a small-bladed knife was inserted just under the skin and, with the blade parallel to the skin, all adhesions between fascia and skin was divided. This was a delicate and time-consuming procedure. When the band had been totally freed it was snapped by forceful extension of the finger. The results were not as satisfactory as with fasciectomy but skin survival was better. As the band had been left in the palm, some form of splintage was necessary for years after the operation.

Recurrence of palmar fibrosis occasionally occurs and it is not unusual for the condition to recur in another finger.

Other deformities of the hand

The deformities of paralysis of the ulnar, median, and radial nerves have been described in Chapter 5 and the student must be able to distinguish them from Dupuytren's contracture.

The wasting of the interossei, particularly the first dorsal interosseus between thumb and index finger, may give a good clue that one is dealing with a patient suffering from ulnar paralysis.

Trigger finger and trigger thumb

In these conditions the patient states that he or she has no difficulty in flexing the finger or thumb but that extension is difficult and, after a feeling of resistance, the digit suddenly straightens with a click.

The pathology of the condition lies in the flexor tendon sheath which has become narrowed for a short part of its length. This narrowing characteristically occurs in front of the metacarpal head. The cause may be non-specific inflammation or rheumatoid disease. It is, in fact, a form of tenosynovitis stenosans.

The explanation of why extension rather than flexion is affected is probably as follows. In flexion, the tendon is under tension and tends to be slightly thinner than in extension. It therefore passes easily through the narrowed segment. In extension, however, it is not under tension and tends to 'bunch up' at the narrowed segment and become obstructed. Eventually the power of the extensors pulls it through the constriction and it is released with a click.

The condition is seen in two main groups of patients—the middle-aged (usually women) and, for some unexplained reason, children during the first year of life. In the latter group it usually affects the thumb and may go on to a complete obstruction to extension. These babies are almost always sent up to hospital with the diagnosis of a 'dislocated thumb'.

Treatment
Surgical excision of part of the circumference of the narrowed segment cures the condition. Occasionally a mild case in an adult can be successfully treated by an injection of hydrocortisone into the affected sheath.

Ganglia of the flexor tendon sheath

Small tense ganglia are sometimes found deep to the flexor crease at the base of a finger. They tend to be painful if the patient carries some heavy object, e.g. a suitcase. They are usually palpable but may be very small.

Treatment is by excision.

INJURIES OF THE HAND AND FINGERS

The hand is the part of the body most prone to injury and for this reason many hospitals have a special hand-injury unit.

Tendon injuries

These are usually the result of industrial accidents but may also be caused by knife wounds and cuts by sharp edges of glass. It is advisable to consider injuries to flexor tendons separately from injuries to extensor tendons.

Division of flexor superficialis and profundus tendons
Throughout most of their length the flexor tendons are surrounded by areolar tissue. Primary repair in these regions give good results. Most surgeons use fine stainless steel wire for the repair and after the operation immobilize the fingers, where tendons have been repaired, in flexion for 2–3 weeks.

There is an area, unfortunately, where the results of primary tendon suture are not satisfactory. This is in that area in which the superficialis and profundus tendons run together through the fibrous tunnel on the flexor aspect of the finger. It extends from the level of the distal palmar crease to the proximal finger flexion crease, i.e. a distance in the adult finger of about two inches. Primary repair of cut tendons in this area leads almost inevitably to adhesion formation between the two tendons and between the tendons and the tunnel or sheath.

For this reason, the primary treatment is limited to debridement of the wound and suture of the skin. As soon as the pain has settled, the patient is encouraged to passively move the finger joints until a full range of movement is achieved.

About 6–8 weeks later, when all inflammation has settled, the cut profundus and sublimis tendons are excised and replaced by a free tendon graft. The donor tendon must be one which the patient does not need: the palmaris longus or the long extensor of the fourth toe. The graft is sutured to the proximal stump of the profundus, which was left when the profundus and sublimis tendons were excised, and to the small remnant which has been left attached to the distal phalanx. Some authorities prefer to 'bury' the distal end of the graft into the distal phalanx and secure it in this position with a suture. Most of the fibrous tunnel is excised, small loops being left through which the graft is threaded and which stop it from bowstringing.

After 2 or 3 weeks of immobilization in the flexed position, active mobilization is commenced. It is important to encourage the patient to move each joint individually.

Division of the superficialis tendon alone
This usually occurs in lacerations over the metacarpo-phalangeal joint and proximal phalanx. Complete division causes loss of active flexion of the proximal interphalangeal joint. This can be diagnosed by asking the patient to flex the p.i.p. joint while the other fingers are held straight. If the superficialis tendon is intact the patient can hold the proximal interphalangeal flexed to 90° with the profundus tendon slack. If the superficialis tendon has been divided the profundus tendon is kept tight to maintain the flexed position of the finger.

As there is usually no significant disability following this injury, no special treatment is advised.

Division of the profundus tendon alone
This occurs in lacerations over the proximal or middle phalanges. It is important to remember that the superficialis tendon splits to allow the profundus tendon to pass through it and that this 'splitting' occurs over the proximal part of the proximal phalanx. A laceration at this level may sever the profundus tendon alone.

Some surgeons favour primary suture of the profundus tendon which has been cut in isolation. Others prefer not to repair it but to advise fusion of the distal interphalangeal joint in about 45° of flexion instead. This results in a good grip and avoids the danger of a stiff finger—particularly stiffness of the proximal interphalangeal joint—which may follow tendon repair.

Division of the tendon of flexor pollicis longus
This tendon is treated in the same way as the profundus tendon in the finger: primary repair is not advised when the division has occurred in the fibrous sheath. There are, however, some cases of division in the distal part of the sheath (over the proximal phalanx) which can be successfully treated by the

procedure named 'advancement'. In this procedure the tendon is lengthened at the level of the lower forearm and then 'advanced' through the sheath for 1–2 cm, and its distal end sutured to a stump of tendon which has been left attached to the distal phalanx. Aftercare is the same as for cut profundus tendons in the fingers.

Division of extensor tendons
The extensor digitorum longus tendons on the back of the hand are surrounded by loose areolar tissue and primary repair is usually successful. The same treatment is applicable to division of the tendon of extensor pollicis longus.

Rupture of extensor pollicis longus tendon
The tendon of extensor pollicis longus may undergo spontaneous rupture resulting in loss of active extension of the interphalangeal joint of the thumb. This is characteristically seen 5–6 weeks after a Colles' fracture when the tendon undergoes attrition and rupture due either to rubbing on the roughened bone or to ischaemia of the tendon.

Repair is often impossible because of the poor condition of the tendon in the region of the rupture. Poor tendon tissue is excised and the distal segment of it is joined to another muscle and tendon which can be diverted from its normal action without incapacitating the patient. The muscle commonly used for this is the extensor carpi radialis longus. Some surgeons use extensor indicis proprius but this is not advised as some interference with m.p. joint extension of the index finger may be caused.

The boutonnière deformity

This consists of a flexion deformity of the proximal interphalangeal joint with a hyperextension deformity of the distal interphalangeal joint. It follows

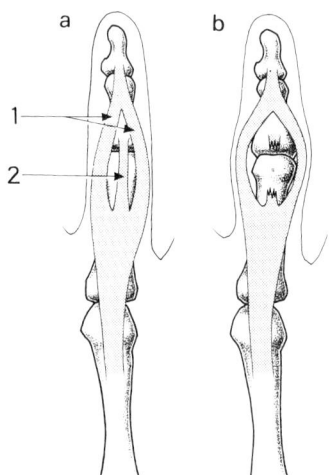

FIG. 24.3. The 'boutonnière' or 'button hole' injury. (a) The normal extensor expansion showing: (1) the lateral slips; (2) the middle slip tear. (b) The middle slip tear.

sudden flexion injuries of the p.i.p. joint as seen, for example, when the finger is hit by a cricket ball. The p.i.p. joint becomes swollen and tender and the swelling usually persists for several weeks, as it subsides the deformity becomes apparent.

The normal extensor expansion of the finger divides into three slips on the dorsal aspect of the proximal phalanx. The central slip crosses the p.i.p. joint and inserts into the base of the middle phalanx. The two lateral slips curve as they pass distally and joint together before inserting into the base of the terminal phalanx. In this injury the central slip becomes detached from the base of the middle phalanx resulting in deficient extension of the joint and the tendency for the head of the proximal phalanx to 'buttonhole' through the extensor expansion (Fig. 24.3). As it does so, the lateral slips tend to act more as flexors than extensors of the p.i.p. joint, thus adding to the deformity. Any attempt at extension is transferred to the distal interphalangeal joint resulting in hyperextension thereof.

Several procedures are advised in the treatment of this condition, but if the function of the fingers is good and the deformity not gross, it is probably best left alone.

Mallet finger

This is a flexion deformity of the distal interphalangeal joint and is seen following flexion injuries, sustained, for example, by women making beds when the finger is caught in a fold in the sheet.

Two types exist:
1. The extensor tendon is avulsed from the dorsal surface of the terminal phalanx. In this type, healing is usually deficient even with adequate splinting and the patient should be warned of the final result—a droop of about 30°.
2. A small fragment of bone is avulsed from the dorsal aspect of the terminal phalanx by the pull of the extensor tendon (Fig. 24.4). The result of treatment in these cases is better because of union of this fragment with the rest of the terminal phalanx.

The finger should be splinted with the distal interphalangeal joint in hyperextension for about 4–6 weeks. Some authorities advise the wearing of a removable splint for a further 6 weeks thereafter.

Division of digital nerves

Digital nerves may be divided at the same time as the flexor tendons or in isolation. Sensory loss along the relevant part of the finger ensues. Treatment

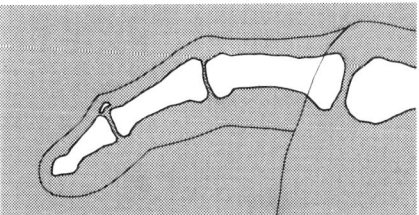

FIG. 24.4. Radiographic appearance of the fracture type of mallet finger.

is by primary suture in clean incised wounds or delayed suture in contaminated wounds. Marking of the nerve ends with black sutures at the time of initial skin closure is advised if secondary repair is contemplated. This facilitates identification of the ends of the nerve.

Nerve suture is relatively simple in the palm where the nerves are large, but difficult in the fingers where they are small. Fine suture material (e.g. 00000 silk) is required.

Fractures of the metacarpals

These are usually due to direct trauma and unless grossly displaced do not require reduction. Union is usually rapid and although some deformity may be evident in the first few months after the fracture, e.g. in the shaft of the index or little finger metacarpals, remoulding is common. Two types of metacarpal fracture deserve special mention.

Fracture of the neck of the fifth metacarpal

This is known as the boxer's fracture and is usually sustained in blows with the clenched fist. The head of the metacarpal becomes angled towards the palm and the degree of final deformity if it is left uncorrected can be gauged by looking at the fist from the distal side and comparing it with the uninjured side. If it is severe the fracture should be reduced and immobilized in a forearm plaster cast extending down to the proximal phalanges. If the deformity is slight the fracture should be treated by early mobilization.

Fracture of the base of the thumb metacarpal

This is a common injury and there is often some angulation into flexion present. Reduction is often difficult and, in fact is not always necessary as the resultant deformity is slight and there is little or no interference with function.

Bennett's fracture–dislocation

This is a fracture–dislocation of the carpo-metacarpal joint of the thumb. There is usually a small triangular fragment from the metacarpal which remains in normal relationship to the trapezium whereas the rest of the metacarpal displaces proximally (Fig. 24.5).

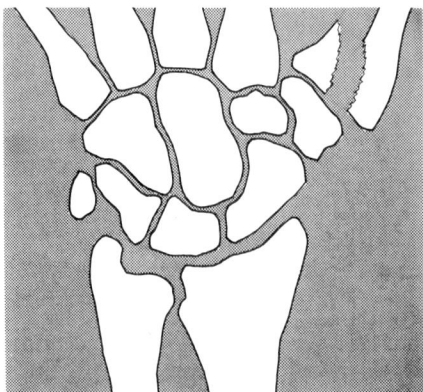

FIG. 24.5. Bennett's fracture–dislocation of the carpo-metacarpal joint of the thumb.

Although the displacement is easy to reduce, the reduction is difficult to hold. Charnley's method of plaster fixation in which the base of the metacarpal is pressed distally and against the carpus while the head of the metacarpal is pressed into extension has been found to be effective but open reduction and internal fixation with Kirschner wires may be necessary. The action of these wires is reinforced by applying a plaster cast, and the cast and the wires are retained for 6 weeks. Thereafter both wires and plaster are removed and active movements started.

Fractures of the phalanges

Fractures of the phalanges should be reduced if angulated or displaced and then immobilized on a malleable finger splint. We prefer to use the 'intrinsic plus' position for immobilization of the finger: 90° flexion at the m.p. joint and extension at the i.p. joints.

Occasionally the fingers have to be held in flexion if a fracture of the proximal phalanx tends to angulate into extension of the distal fragment. The danger of stiffness of the proximal interphalangeal joint must always be kept in mind and mobilization started as soon as the fracture has united.

Undisplaced fractures of the phalanges may be treated by strapping the injured finger to the next one and encouraging early movement. Fractures into a joint with disruption of the joint surface may require open reduction and immobilization by transfixion using Kirschner wires. Again, early mobilization is beneficial.

Dislocations of finger and thumb joints

Most dislocations of metacarpo-phalangeal and interphalangeal joints are simple to reduce, with the exception of the interphalangeal joint of the thumb. The flexor pollicis longus tendon often becomes displaced and lies between the dislocated phalanges: open reduction is then necessary.

Mobilization should be begun after a few days in simple dislocations and in 7–10 days after an open reduction has been carried out.

Sprains of collateral ligaments

The collateral ligaments of the metacarpo-phalangeal joints are prone to sprains and tears, particularly in sporting injuries. Most cause pain for several months particularly when stretched. The medial collateral ligament of the m.p. joint of the thumb may be torn and, if it is not treated, may lead to permanent weakness and an increased range of abduction of the thumb. Operative repair may be necessary if the disability is serious.

RECOMMENDATIONS FOR FURTHER READING

PULVERTAFT, R. G. (1965) Problems of flexor tendon surgery of the hand, *J. Bone Jt Surg.* **47A**, 123–32.

RANG, M. (1966) Dupuytrens contracture, original description. In *Anthology of Orthopaedics*, pp. 109–14. E. & S. Livingstone. Edinburgh.

RANG, M. (1966) Bennett's fracture, original description. In *Anthology of Orthopaedics*, pp. 95–6. E. & S. Livingstone, Edinburgh.

RANK, B. K., WAKEFIELD, A. R., and HEUSTON, J. T. (1973) *The Surgery of Repair as Applied to Hand Injuries* (4th edn), Churchill–Livingstone, Edinburgh.

25 The hip region

ANATOMY AND DEVELOPMENT

The hip is a ball-and-socket joint. The socket is called the acetabulum (Latin for 'vinegar bowl'), and the ball is formed by the femoral capital epiphysis in children and in adults by the head of the femur.

The acetabulum develops in cartilage which is ossified from three primary centres—those for the ilium, ischium, and pubis. The advancing edges of these areas of ossification meet in the base of the acetabulum leaving, during growth, the triradiate cartilage. This is an important point and is used in measuring the acetabular angles.

The epiphysis of the head of the femur usually begins to ossify during the fourth, fifth, or sixth month of life. This means that the diagnosis of dislocations and subluxations of the hip joint are difficult to make before the fourth month of life, as radiographs do not show the position of the ossification centre for the capital epiphysis and hence the position of the cartilaginous head of the femur is difficult to gauge.

There is also a separate epiphysis for the greater trochanter whose ossific nucleus appears at approximately 4 years. Development of the upper end of the femur and hence its definitive shape depends on the relative rate of growth of the metaphyses opposite these two epiphyses.

There are two angles of clinical importance in the upper femur, and they are both between the neck and the shaft of the femur.

If the neck–shaft angle is viewed from the anterior aspect (actually slightly lateral of anterior, i.e. at right-angles to the neck) the angle between the neck and the shaft will be seen to be approximately 120°. This is called the angle of inclination, and the normal range in the adult is 120–140° (Fig. 25.1).

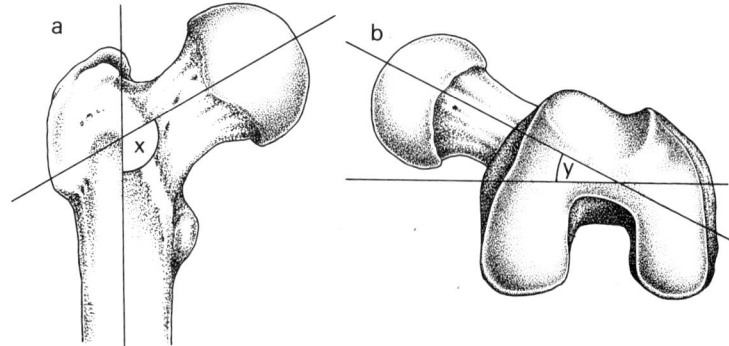

FIG. 25.1. (a) The upper end of the femur showing the angle of inclination (x). (b) The femur as seen from the lower end showing the angle of anteversion (y).

If the upper shaft is viewed from its true lateral aspect—which can be ascertained by looking at the femoral condyles—it will be noted that the neck of the femur is turned forwards a few degrees from the coronal plane. This is called the angle of anteversion and varies at different ages. It is greatest in the newborn and diminishes with age. If the normal moulding forces which occur with growth are interfered with in any way, as in congenital dislocation of the hip, the angle may not diminish with increasing age.

CONGENITAL AND DEVELOPMENTAL ANOMALIES OF THE HIP

The hips of newborn infants are remarkably mobile. The capsule and muscles are lax and allow the hip to be flexed, abducted, adducted, and rotated through a very wide range of movements. During the first 10 days of life this range of movement diminishes. Normally the diminution affects both hips to the same extent.

Clunking hips

If one examines the hips of newborn infants routinely, one sometimes finds that it is possible to dislocate one or both of them. The common method to demonstrate that the hip is dislocatable is to flex it to 90°, adduct it to neutral and then gently press the head of the femur backwards into the buttock. The head will then be felt to click over the posterior rim of the acetabulum.

If the thigh is then abducted (the hip still being in the 90°-flexed position) the head of the femur will be felt to 'click' or 'clunk' forwards into the socket (acetabulum) and redislocation is impossible unless the femur is once more adducted (Fig. 25.2). A hip demonstrating this phenomenon is referred to as a 'congenitally dislocatable hip' (CDH), or in local parlance a 'clunking' hip.

If the capsule is allowed to tighten with the hip in the dislocated position, reduction becomes increasingly difficult with the passage of time, and one is then faced with an irreducably dislocated hip.

If the capsule tightens with the hip in the reduced position the hip usually develops normally and in the majority of cases ceases to be dislocatable. In a small number of cases, however, dislocation remains possible.

The object of management of these 'clunking hips' is to keep the hip reduced

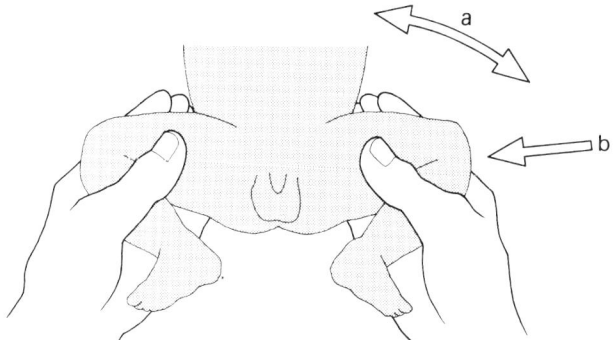

FIG. 25.2. The 'clunking' test for instability of the hip. (a) Abduction–adduction range. (b) Direction of pressure.

until the danger of dislocation has passed. This is achieved by holding the hip in full abduction and flexed to 90°. This is referred to as the 90–90 frog position. During the first few months of life this can be achieved by applying the nappies in such a manner that the baby is unable to adduct the thighs to any extent. As a large bulk of nappy is required, the mother is advised to use two nappies instead of one. As the child grows this method often becomes less successful and the mother is then advised to apply a plastic 'over nappy' or Craig splint.

This splint is made of firm sheet plastic and provides a more efficient method of holding the hips abducted. It is worn over a single nappy. In this way the hip is kept in its safe position of abduction.

It is our practice to examine these children regularly to be sure that the hip is remaining in the reduced position. The child is seen every 3–4 weeks. Most clunking hips cease to be dislocatable by the third month.

At 6 months the hips are X-rayed, and if the radiograph shows a good capital epiphysis and satisfactory acetabular development, the splint is removed or, if the child is in double nappies, they may be reduced to a single nappy. If, however, there is any doubt about the epiphyseal or acetabular development the hips are kept in the 90–90 frog position until development is considered adequate.

Clicking hips

In addition to the dislocatable or 'clunking' hips there are a large number of babies referred to the orthopaedic clinic with 'clicking' hips. We use this term to describe those hips which can be felt or heard to click on movement but which do not exhibit any tendency to dislocate. It must be appreciated that some clinics use this term to describe all hips which click or clunk.

We feel that it is worthwhile to follow these children as well through the first 6 months or so of life, i.e. until the radiograph shows satisfactory capital epiphyses in satisfactory acetabula. They are examined once a month and the mothers encouraged to use double nappies. The vast majority of these children develop normal hips but a definite percentage do not develop normally.

The earliest sign that development is not proceeding normally is that the range of abduction in flexion of the hip becomes restricted. If this restriction of abduction is allowed to progress there is a danger of the capital epiphysis dislocating posteriorly from the acetabulum.

For this reason any restriction of abduction is considered a definite indication for the application of a Craig splint. The effect of this is to stretch the adductors, a process which may take a few weeks. Once abduction to 90° has been regained development progresses normally.

If abduction remains restricted it is our practice to examine the child under an anaesthetic and if the adductors remain tight, to perform a subcutaneous tenotomy of the adductor origin and then immobilize the hips in the 90–90 frog position in a plaster of Paris cast. Tenotomy of the adductors often reveals that the hip is, in fact, dislocatable or subluxatable.

Once the child is in a 'frog' plaster it follows a routine of 3-monthly plaster changes with radiographs being taken when the old plaster has been removed. From these radiographs the development of the capital epiphysis and the acetabulum is assessed.

When development is considered adequate the plaster fixation is changed

The hip region

to an intermediate position of 45° abduction and flexion for a few months before being discontinued completely.

Ortolani's test
This test is widely used in the early diagnosis of 'clunking' hips and is based on the fact that the hip reduces as the flexed thigh is abducted. The examiner holds the thigh between fingers and thumb and with the hips and knees flexed to 90° gently abducts the thigh from the 'knees-together' position to full abduction. If the hip is in the dislocated position the examiner encounters slight resistance to abduction followed by a clunk as the head rides forward into the acetabulum. This is referred to as 'Ortolani's click of reduction'. If the thigh is then adducted again the head dislocates over the posterior rim of the acetabulum: 'Ortolani's click of dislocation'.

Radiographs
These are taken at birth or at the first visit to the clinic. Gross dislocation of the hip may be obvious but minor displacements may be difficult to assess because the capital epiphysis is not visible and the acetabulum is poorly identified. Two special views are occasionally taken.

1. *Shenton's line.* If the legs are held together and the hips extended when the radiograph is taken it is possible on the radiograph to trace the line of the undersurface of the neck which when continued in the form of an arc is continuous with the undersurface of the superior pubic ramus. Shenton's line is broken in CDH (Fig. 25.3).

2. *Von Rosen's lines.* If a radiograph is taken with the legs each abducted 45°, i.e. total of 90° abduction, lines may be drawn on the radiograph along the shaft of the femur and produced upwards to cut the pelvis. These are Von Rosen's lines. It may be obvious that one line is in a more cranial position than the other. In normal hips this line should pass below the anterior inferior iliac spine.

Diagnosis in late cases
Diagnosis in children over the age of 6 months is usually relatively easy.

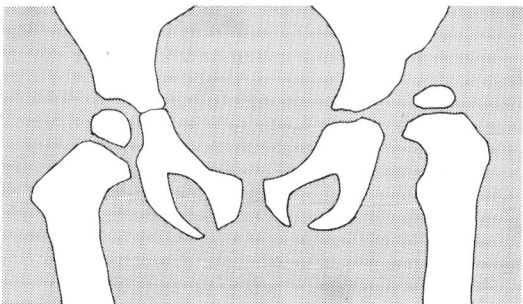

FIG. 25.3. Radiographic appearance of a case of left-sided congenital dislocation of the hip showing Shenton's line intact on the right and broken on the left. Note also that the left acetabulum is dysplastic.

Abduction of the hip is reduced and the classical signs of congenital dislocation are present: the affected lower limb is shorter, the skin creases are asymmetrical and 'telescoping' of the thigh may be elicitable.

Treatment of late cases
Treatment consists of reduction, which is usually preceded by traction to allow the head of the femur to come down to the level of the acetabulum, followed by plaster fixation until development is adequate. The time taken for development is longer in cases diagnosed late. Closed reduction may be impossible due to the presence of soft tissue in the acetabulum or to tightness of the ligaments and capsule and in these cases open reduction is required. Some authorities follow the open reduction with a corrective de-rotation osteotomy of the femur to reduce the anteversion deformity at the upper end of the femur which usually accompanies the dislocation of the hip. This is usually done about 6 weeks after the open reduction.

Diagnosis and treatment after walking has commenced
It is relatively rare now for a patient with a dislocated hip to present for the first time over the age of 1 year (the approximate age at which children begin to walk). In these cases the child walks with a Trendelenberg 'lurch' and the Trendelenberg sign is positive. If both hips are dislocated the child walks with a 'rolling-sailor gait', swinging the shoulders to each side as he or she takes weight on the corresponding leg.

Treatment is again by traction followed by manipulative reduction, or if impossible, by open reduction. The chances of obtaining a normal hip after treatment diminish as the age of the child increases and most authorities feel that the indication for reduction diminishes as the child approaches the age of 4 years. Congenitally dislocated hips usually have a wide range of movement and as age progresses the danger of a stiff hip after reduction increases. This is a particular danger in a child with bilateral dislocations. It is not unusual for one hip to become stiff after treatment and for the other to be normal so that the child ends up with one mobile and one stiff hip—a condition considered by many to be less desirable than two mobile but dislocated hips. For this reason the upper age limit for bilateral cases is lower than for unilateral cases.

Acetabular dysplasia
By this term we mean that the development of the acetabulum is deficient. In young babies it can be diagnosed by measuring the 'acetabular angle'. This is the angle the roof of the acetabulum makes with the horizontal and is measured on an antero-posterior radiograph of the pelvis by drawing a line through the centre of the Y-shaped cartilage in the floor of the acetabulum and measuring the angle made with this line by a second line drawn from the base of the acetabulum where it is cut by the horizontal line to the outer lip of the acetabulum. In acetabular dysplasia this angle is increased.

Although usually seen in dislocated hips, acetabular dysplasia may occur with a normally placed capital epiphysis. The effect of this dysplasia is that as the child gets older the head of the femur tends to slip outwards and upwards (subluxation).

The dysplasia may be treated in the very young by encouraging development by means of frog plaster. In older patients treatment may be by operative reconstruction of the acetabulum as seen in the arthroplasties of Salter and Chiari, in which the shape of the side wall of the pelvis is altered to increase the 'cover' of the head, or in the shelf operation, in which the upper part of the acetabulum is extended laterally by 'turning down' some of the outer cortex of the ilium and securing it in this position by packing bone grafts between it and the remaining ilium.

It should be mentioned that all the above abnormal developments of the hip are commoner in girls than boys—a fact that has never been satisfactorily explained.

CLINICAL CONDITIONS OF THE HIP

Septic arthritis of the hip in infancy

This condition is given special consideration, mainly because of its catastrophic effects on the head of the femur. If an infant develops septic arthritis it is highly likely that the capital epiphysis will be infarcted and may well sequestrate. These children present with a high temperature, a high white cell count, and a positive blood culture—if one is fortunate enough to obtain a specimen of blood before antibiotic treatment is started.

The hip joint becomes very irritable, but this is difficult to diagnose in an infant because of the difficulties of communication. For this reason, these children are often diagnosed late and when surgical drainage of the hip is carried out, the head of the femur has already become necrotic. For this reason, early diagnosis and early decompression of the hip are essential and the avoidance of necrosis of the head of the femur. The condition is also known as 'Tom Smith's arthritis' after the author of the original description.

Perthes' disease

Perthes' disease is an osteochondritis of the capital epiphysis of the femur. It occurs more commonly in boys than girls and usually affects children of 5–10 years. Children presenting for the first time with hip troubles tend to fall into three age groups. Those between the ages of 0 and 5 years old are usually suffering from CDH or its complications; from 5 to 10 years from Perthes' disease; and from 10 to 15 years from displacement of the upper femoral epiphysis. Infections and trauma, of course, affect any age group.

Symptoms
The child presents with one of two symptoms: either he has pain in the hip or the parents have noticed a limp.

On examination, most children with Perthes' disease exhibit the findings which are grouped together under the heading of 'irritable hip'. By this is meant a hip which is painful and which on attempted movement exhibits spasm of the surrounding muscle. The limp of which these children complain is of the antalgic type, the child hurrying off the more painful hip, so that the walking cycle is unevenly distributed, more time being spent on the good hip, less time on the painful hip. Remember that hip conditions may give rise to pain felt in the knee.

Radiographs
These are of particular interest in Perthes' disease. There is a cycle of changes which usually takes 18–24 months to be completed. The capital epiphysis at

172 *Orthopaedics for Undergraduates*

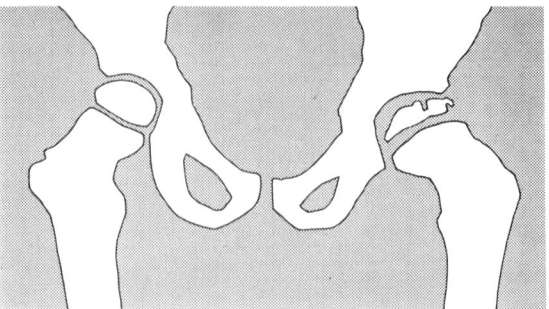

FIG. 25.4. Radiographic appearance of Perthes' disease of the left hip.

first becomes dense, then becomes fragmented, and then gradually returns to normal. It is, of course, often difficult to decide on one radiograph to which point in the cycle the disease has progressed.

The shape of the capital epiphysis may become distorted and if this occurs, the head is usually permanently flattened. There are also X-ray changes occurring in the neck of the femur. The neck may show the presence of cysts and inevitably widens so that the diameter of the neck, as seen on the anteroposterior radiographs, is greater than on the normal side (Fig. 25.4).

Pathology

The cause of these changes is not certain. Since they can be produced in experimental animals by occluding the blood to the capital epiphysis, it is supposed that it is a vascular phenomenon. What is believed to be occurring is virtually an infarction of the capital epiphysis followed by revascularization.

Treatment

There is great debate as to the best method of treatment of these children. Opinion varies from the school which keeps the child off the hip during the whole cycle, to the school which does not restrict the activity of the child in any way. All schools agree that during the irritable stage the hip should be immobilized, and the easiest way to achieve this is to put the leg on traction with the child in bed. It is also felt that the chances of recovery with a normal-shaped femoral head are probably increased if weight bearing is restricted and if the hip is kept in some degree of abduction to improve containment. For this reason, children are initially treated in abduction plasters, usually of the 'broomstick' variety, and later allowed to get about on a pattern-ended caliper, which is an overlong caliper fixed to a separate sole a few inches below the shoe so that the child's foot is about 10–15 cm off the ground. The other shoe has to be raised an equal amount to allow the child to walk. This restriction of weight bearing is continued until the cycle of changes in the femoral capital epiphysis is complete.

Some authorities suggest osteotomy of the upper end of the femur or of the acetabulum to increase the degree of containment of the head of the femur. At present this is not done in our department.

Prognosis
Clinical studies spread over many years have established that the prognosis for recovery both as regards stiffness and pain is good. The factor which affects recovery most is the age of onset of the disease: the earlier the onset, the better the prognosis.

Irritable hip

This term is used to define a clinical entity of a painful hip with spasm of surrounding muscle on attempted movement. During the course of a year, some 70–100 children are admitted under this diagnosis to the Royal Liverpool Children's Hospital. It is a blanket diagnosis and implies that further investigation is necessary. These children are admitted and kept in bed on traction while the investigations proceed.

Investigations done are a 4-hourly estimation of the temperature and pulse rate of the child, estimation of the white cell count, the latex fixation test, the serum uric acid, and ESR. Virus studies may be carried out if considered relevant. Some children are found to be suffering from such conditions as osteomyelitis of the ilium or neck of the femur, septic arthritis of the hip, Perthes' disease, or tuberculous infections. When all of these diagnoses have been ruled out the child is diagnosed—by exclusion—to have been suffering from transient synovitis of the hip. In these cases, the symptoms rapidly resolve and the physical signs disappear. This is a common finding in irritable hips, but all children with irritable hips must be screened as this could be the first clue to a condition such as Perthes' disease.

Slipping of the upper femoral epiphysis

The epiphyseal cartilage of the upper end of the femur becomes displaced in some children. It should be remembered that the epiphysis itself stays in the acetabulum so that the displacement is more of the femoral metaphysis on the epiphysis than a slipping of the femoral epiphysis as the name implies.

When severe, the displacement is such that the neck of the femur turns forwards and passes upwards or, to describe the displacement in the conventional manner, the capital epiphysis comes to lie behind and slightly below its normal attachment to the neck (Fig. 25.5).The condition occurs more in boys than girls and normally between the ages of 10 and 15 years. Classically, it occurs in overweight children, and is said to occur in those with delayed onset of puberty.

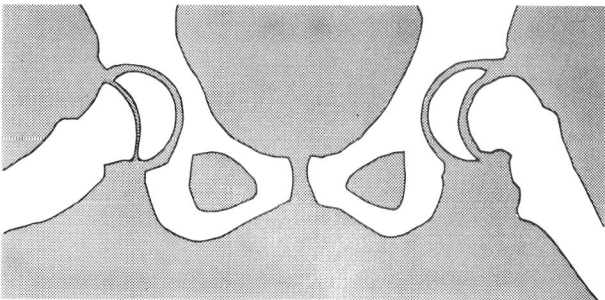

FIG. 25.5. Slipping of the upper femoral epiphysis.

The hip may be irritable or painful or the site of deformity and the patient may give the history of an accident at the outset of symptoms. There are three main types of displacement: (1) the chronic, in which symptoms have been present for several months; (2) the acute, which is usually seen as a traumatic episode, e.g. the child falls off his bicycle or out of a tree; and (3) the acute-on-chronic in which the child has had some aching in the hip for some months and then undergoes a traumatic episode which aggravates the symptoms. The pain may be felt in the hip or in the knee. This is another example of referred pain and is due to the fact that the hip and knee share a nerve supply from the femoral and obturator nerves.

Clinical findings
The child in the acute stage may have an irritable hip. In cases with severe displacement the leg will be noted to be lying in external rotation and if the hip is flexed the knee instead of passing upwards to the chest passes upwards and outwards towards the shoulder or axilla. The range of movement is restricted in the acute phase and in the chronic phase it will be noted that the range of rotation has moved into the external segment and it may not be possible to internally rotate the hip beyond the neutral position. The child may have a positive Trendelenberg sign. There may be true shortening of the limb, and there may be an adduction deformity.

Treatment
In the acute and the acute-on-chronic types, an attempt is made to reduce the displacement by gentle manipulation. It is usually impossible to reduce the hip in the acute-on-chronic type to a position better than it had been before the acute episode. The diagnosis of this slip and of the degree of correction is best made by studying the lateral radiograph of the hip. If the displacement in the chronic type or in the other types after reduction is such that less than one-third of the metaphysis is uncovered, it is customary for an attempt to be made to fix the epiphysis in this position by internal fixation using Moore's pins. Following this the patient is treated recumbent and then ambulant with protection until the epiphyseal line has closed. This normally occurs within 6 months of operation. If, however, the displacement after reduction or in the chronic case is more than one-third of the width of the metaphysis, as seen in the lateral radiograph, it is customary to leave the epiphysis in this position and allow it to unite to the shaft. Corrective osteotomy is then done at the level of, or just above, the lesser trochanter. During the time of waiting for the epiphysis to unite to the metaphysis, the child is treated on traction in internal rotation to prevent further displacement.

Any forceful attempt at reduction may damage the blood-supply of the epiphysis and lead to avascular necrosis.

Coxa vara
If the angle of inclination of the neck of the femur (the angle between the neck and shaft of the femur as seen from the front) is less than 120°, the condition of coxa vara is said to be present. The causes of coxa vara have been arranged, for convenience, into categories depending on the level at which they are acting. Conditions in childhood may lead to development of coxa vara in the adult as may conditions coming on later in life. The classification is as follows:

1. Conditions affecting the epiphysis:
   (a) septic arthritis of the hip in infancy;
   (b) Perthes' disease;
   (c) avascular necrosis of the head of the femur.
2. Conditions affecting the epiphyseal line:
   (a) slipping of the upper femoral epiphysis;
   (b) congenital coxa vara (see below).
3. Conditions affecting the neck of the femur: fractures; infections; tumours; rickets; and Paget's disease.
4. Conditions affecting the trochanteric region: fractures; infections; tumours; rickets; and Paget's disease.

Congenital coxa vara
This is an interesting but rare condition in which the development of the upper end of the femur is deficient in such a way as to allow the angle of inclination to diminish. Early attempts at explanation were made difficult because of the presence of large numbers of patients suffering from rickets. The condition of congenital coxa vara is now known to be separate from these and can be distinguished from them by the presence of an abnormal epiphyseal line on X-ray which, instead of being a single plate, develops the shape of an inverted V or Y, so that there is a small triangular island of ossified cartilage seen on the undersurface of the neck in the antero-posterior view (Fig. 25.6). With continuing development, the capital epiphysis comes to lie further and further down the shaft of the femur and the greater trochanter tends to bend over towards the hip joint.

In early life the diagnosis may be confused with congenital dislocation of the hip. The perineum is wide. Abduction of the affected hip is restricted and the child walks with a Trendelenberg lurch. The diagnosis is usually apparent on X-ray, and as growth continues the loss of abduction becomes more and more of a problem. Treatment depends on the severity of the condition and if severe, abduction osteotomy in the intertrochanteric region is the method of choice.

Osteoarthritis of the hip joint

In our department, the hip joint is probably the joint most commonly found to be affected with degenerative arthritis. Patients are usually middle-aged or elderly and present with symptoms of pain and/or stiffness. The pain is felt in the groin, buttock, or over the greater trochanter, and the stiffness often first

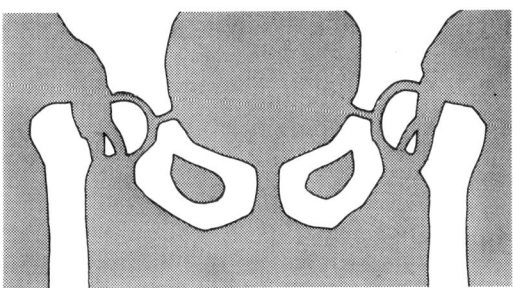

FIG. 25.6. Bilateral congenital coxa vara.

becomes apparent when the patient tries to tie his shoe laces or to lift the foot on to the platform of a bus.

Characteristically the degenerative hip assumes a position of progressive deformity into adduction, flexion, and external rotation. The degree of adduction can be assessed by measuring the true and apparent lengths of the leg. If there is apparent shortening greater than true shortening, the hip lies in adduction. The patient himself may draw your attention to this by stating that if he stands with his legs parallel (the normal procedure) the foot on the affected side does not reach the ground. This is the explanation of the term 'apparent shortening' of the limb.

Types of osteoarthritis of the hip
It is customary to describe two types of osteoarthritis of the hip joint:
1. *Primary.* This comes on for no obvious reason and with no obvious predisposing cause.
2. *Secondary.* This comes on after some condition which has rendered the articular surfaces of the hip joint irregular. Examples of such conditions are septic arthritis, fractures, Perthes' disease, CDH, slipping of the upper femoral epiphysis, and rheumatoid disease. Rheumatoid disease is a very common cause of secondary osteoarthritis of the hip joint.

Clinical findings
The patient walks with a limp. Both the Trendelenberg lurch and the shortening may contribute towards the limp. The hip has a restricted range of movement, particularly of rotation, and the limb may be found to be lying in adduction, flexion (as shown by Thomas's hip flexion test), and external rotation.

Radiographs
These show the four classical signs:
(1) loss of joint space;
(2) presence of osteophytes;
(3) presence of sclerosis in the adjacent parts of the bones; and
(4) cyst formation in the head of the femur and the acetabulum.

Treatment
Mild cases respond to conservative treatment which consists of (1) analgesics, (2) restricting the range of movement of the joint by raising the heel of the shoe, (3) restricting the demands on the joint by the use of a walking stick in the opposite hand, and (4) the use of heat in the form of short-wave diathermy, usually associated with mobilization exercises.

If the patient does not respond to this treatment, which must be given for several months before the decision is made, operation may be indicated. There are three operations done for degenerative change in the hip.

1. *Arthrodesis.* In this operation the hip is stiffened by allowing bone to grow across the joint space. This should only be carried out in patients with good movement in the contralateral hip and good movement in the lumbar spine. This is because the movement of the hip which has been fused has to be replaced by a movement of the pelvis. This entails extra movement of the lumbar spine and the fulcrum for this movement is the contralateral hip joint. Arthrodesis, therefore, is usually done only in young people.

2. *Osteotomy.* It was fortuitously discovered that osteotomy of the upper end of the femur relieved the pain of osteoarthritis of the hip. The operation was described by Professor McMurray of Liverpool in 1930 (see Fig. 10.2, p. 54). The mechanism by which this operation relieves the pain is unknown. The effect on the range of movement is unpredictable: in some patients complete fusion of the hip occurs, whereas in others an increased range of movement occurs. The operation, as originally described, entailed external fixation of the hip by means of a plaster of Paris hip spica for 3 months. The use of internal fixation has reduced the time which the patient spends in hospital, but the plaster spica method of fixation is still used in young patients.

3. *Arthoplasty.* Interest over the last 10 years has been focused on the question of replacing the hip joint. One of the early methods was the excision of the head and neck of the femur with the development of a fibrous joint. This was known as the Girdlestone arthroplasty and is now used mainly as a salvage procedure. The hip loses its stability and the patient is virtually certain to require the use of a walking-stick. Other forms of arthroplasty include a cup replacement of the acetabulum (Smith–Peterson); the replacement of the head of the femur with a metal head (Moore or Thompson prosthesis); the replacement of both the acetabulum and the head of the femur by metal (Ring or McKee–Farrar prosthesis; see Fig. 10.3, p. 54), and finally the replacement of the acetabulum by a plastic cup and the head of the femur by a metal prosthesis (Charnley prosthesis; see Fig. 10.3, p. 54). Each method has its advantages and disadvantages. The results are very encouraging and the operation is gaining in popularity.

INJURIES IN THE HIP REGION

Fractures of the acetabulum

The rim of the acetabulum may be fractured as part of a fracture–dislocation of the hip joint when the head of the femur is displaced backwards (see below).

The floor of the acetabulum is fractured by a compressive force acting along the line of the neck of the femur. This injury is seen in patients who fall on to their hips, or in pedestrians knocked down from the side by motor vehicles. Several degrees of injury are seen, ranging from a crack of the acetabular floor to complete medial displacement of the acetabulum and the contained femoral head. This injury is often referred to (wrongly) as a central dislocation of the hip—a better term is 'stove-in hip' or 'stove-in pelvis'.

The treatment of these injuries in this country is usually conservative. The minor degrees of injury do not require reduction and are treated by bed-rest with or without traction until the fracture has united.

In the severe 'stove-in' injuries, reduction by means of longitudinal or lateral traction on the femur is attempted. As in the case of the comminuted vertical compression fracture–dislocations of the ankle, the intention is to realign the joint surfaces in as near an anatomical position as possible accepting that degenerative arthrosis of the joint will probably occur later and further treatment will be necessary. Open reduction of the stove-in hip at the time of injury is a hazardous procedure because of bleeding from the vessels lining the pelvis, and is not recommended. Traction is continued until union has occurred.

Dislocation of the hip joint

As mentioned above these are usually posterior displacements of the head of the femur and may be associated with fractures of the rim of the acetabulum. The common method of production of these injuries is a force applied head-on to the lower end of the femur when the patient is sitting. They are therefore common in motor-car and motor-cycle injuries. The dislocation of the hip may go unnoticed in a patient who has severe injuries to the knee or tibia following a motor-cycle injury and it is therefore a rule in accident units that the hips should always be examined and X-rayed in all severe lower limb injuries. The problem is often made more difficult when the patient is unconscious from a head injury.

Damage to the sciatic nerve often accompanies dislocations of the hip and the neurological state of the limb should be carefully assessed before reduction is attempted.

Treatment is by manipulative reduction under general anaesthesia. Powerful traction may be required. If there is a large posterior acetabular fragment present the reduction may not be stable to compression and open reduction and internal fixation by screws may be necessary.

In either case post-operative traction is applied to the limb until the capsule and ligaments have reconstituted.

The presence of a sciatic paralysis is considered by some authorities to be an indication for open reduction. Most surgeons reduce the dislocation and then await recovery of the nerve.

Fractures of the upper end of the femur

These injuries occur mainly in the elderly and are more common in women than men. The fractures occur either in the neck or in the trochanteric region (Fig. 25.7). They can therefore be called cervical or trochanteric fractures and, since the capsule of the hip joint attaches to the femur just at the junction of the neck and trochanters, are also referred to as intracapsular and extracapsular fractures.

Trochanteric fractures
These occur in an area of good blood-supply and non-union is virtually unheard of. The problems associated with these fractures are: (a) the general

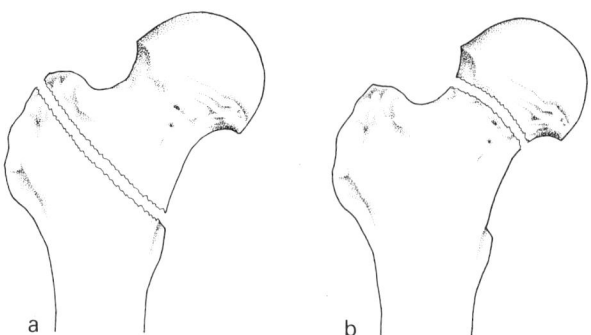

FIG. 25.7. Fractures of the upper end of the femur. (a) Trochanteric region. (b) Cervical region.

effects they have on elderly patients causing immobility with the dangers of deep venous thrombosis and bronchopneumonia; and (b) the tendency for the fracture to angulate into varus after reduction. Both of these problems are fairly successfully solved by early internal fixation by means of a strong pin and plate and then active mobilization of the patient.

Cervical fractures
These carry a poor prognosis for union, especially if they are displaced.

The blood-vessels supplying the head of the femur pass up on the surface of the neck (particularly on the posterior aspect) and are bound down to the neck by the synovium of the hip joint. Any fracture in this area will damage these vessels and endanger the viability of the head of the femur. Aseptic necrosis of the head of the femur is therefore a common complication of these fractures especially those occurring just under the head (the subcapital type). Debility and senility also militate against a successful outcome in these injuries and early internal fixation and rehabilitation is again indicated. It is common practice to use pin and plate fixation for these fractures as well.

If the fracture is grossly displaced and the patient over 65 years of age, many surgeons conclude that the head of the femur will not survive and immediate prosthetic replacement is carried out.

Fracture of the neck of the femur in children

Fortunately these are rare. The fracture is usually in the cervical region and the rate of non-union is high. Internal fixation by means of several fine pins (to minimize trauma to the epiphyseal plate) is the method of treatment most favoured although many cases are treated by manipulation and external fixation by means of a Thomas splint, a frame, or a plaster of Paris spica.

RECOMMENDATIONS FOR FURTHER READING

BARNES, R. (1967) Fracture of the neck of the femur. *J. Bone Jt Surg.* **49B**, 607–17.
GARDEN, R. S. (1971) Malreduction and avascular necrosis in subcapital fractures of the femur. *J. Bone Jt Surg.* **63B**, 183–97.
MCKIBBIN, B. and RALIS, Z. (1974) Pathological changes in a case of Perthes' disease, *J. Bone Jt Surg.* **56B**, 438–47.
RANG, M. (1966) Tom Smith's arthritis of the hip of infants, original description. In *Anthology of Orthopaedics*, pp. 16–17, E. & S. Livingstone, Edinburgh.
RANG, M. (1966) Thomas's hip flexion test, original description. In *Anthology of Orthopaedics*, pp. 137–8, E. & S. Livingstone, Edinburgh.
RATCLIFFE, A. H. C. (1967) Perthes' disease. A study of thirty-four hips observed for 30 years, *J. Bone Jt Surg.* **49B**, 102–7.
SOMERVILLE, E. W. (1967) Results of treating of 100 congenitally dislocated hips, *J. Bone Jt Surg.* **49B**, 258–67.

26 The thigh

Congenital shortening of the femur

The femur is one of the bones more commonly affected by hypoplasia. Usually the whole bone is affected (Fig. 26.1) but occasionally there is, in addition to the shortening, deformity, or absence of the head and neck. The common deformity encountered is coxa vara (see p. 175).
Minor degrees of shortening are treated by leg equalization. More severe degrees are treated by amputation of the limb and subsequent fitting of a prosthesis.

Rupture of the rectus femoris
Spontaneous rupture of the rectus femoris is seen in sports injuries. It is usually due to sudden unpremeditated contraction of the muscle. The patient experience sudden pain, the thigh becomes painful and swollen, and, during the ensuing weeks, a swelling becomes palpable on the anterior aspect of the thigh whenever the quadriceps is contracted. Most patients suffer no disability following this injury and repair is not usually advised.

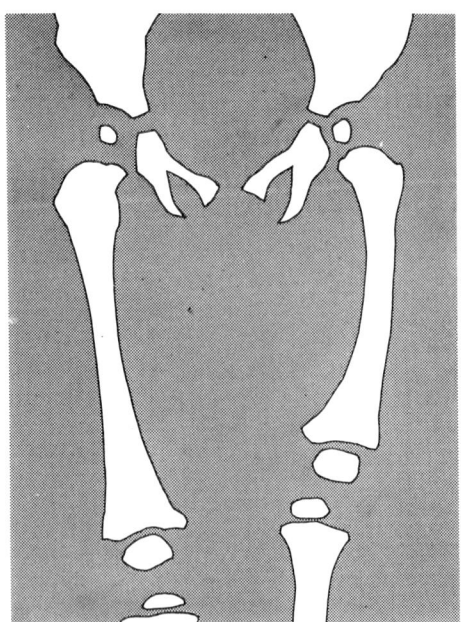

FIG. 26.1. Congenital short femur.

Fractures of the femoral shaft

Most of these fractures are due to direct violence. As the femur lies deep in the thigh surrounded on all sides by vascular muscle, ischaemia of the bone-ends is relatively rare so that delayed union, if it occurs, is more likely to be due to inadequate fixation than to ischaemia.

Mal-union, on the other hand, is relatively common and consists of either angulation or overlapping of the fragments with resultant shortening of the limb. The average adult, however, can easily adapt for shortening of the lower limb of up to 2 cm without developing a limp.

Treatment

Reduction. This is usually achieved by manipulation and traction. Failure to reduce by manipulation is often due to interposition of soft tissues between the bone ends and is an indication for open reduction. End-to-end apposition of the fragments ('hitching') is desirable but not essential.

Immobilization. This is achieved by traction. By applying a gentle pull on the lower fragment, tension is produced in the muscles which cross the fracture line, namely, the quadriceps and hamstrings. The tension in these muscles tends to mould the fragments back into correct alignment. It is important that the tension should be maintained until union of the fracture has occurred.

There are two main methods of applying traction to the femur. The first is by lowering the head of the bed so that the patient lies on an inclined plane with his feet higher than his head and then pulling on the affected leg by means of a weight and pulley device attached to the leg—usually to a metal pin inserted into the upper tibia. The weight provides the traction and the patient's own body weight provides the counter-traction because the patient tends to slide down the inclined plane towards the head of the bed. This method is called 'sliding traction' because the whole system can move back and forth.

The second method of applying traction to the femur is called 'fixed traction' and involves the use of a Thomas splint (Fig. 26.2). In the setting up of this method the patient's lower limb is passed through the ring at the upper end of the Thomas splint and the ring moved up the leg and thigh until it comes to lie against the ischial tuberosity—the lowest point of the pelvis and the part of the bone used to taking weight when a person is sitting.

Traction is now applied to the leg and thigh distal to the fracture. This is done by attaching two strips of adhesive strapping to the sides of the thigh and calf and holding them in position with crêpe bandages. These strips of strapping have tapes attached to their lower ends. The ends of these tapes are tied, under tension, to the cross-piece at the lower end of the Thomas splint.

In this method, the traction is maintained by the tightness of the tapes. The point of counter-traction is where the ring of the splint presses onto the ischial tuberosity. Since nothing moves in this system it is referred to as fixed traction.

Our present practice is to use fixed traction with one modification. It is sometimes found that patients complain of pain at the point of pressure of the ring on the ischial tuberosity, and this pressure can be reduced by pulling the whole splint towards the foot of the bed. Since the fixed traction tapes are attached to the cross-piece of the splint, pulling on the splint does not reduce the traction on the fracture. Traction is applied to the splint either by attaching a weight and pulley arrangement to it, or by tying the end of the splint to

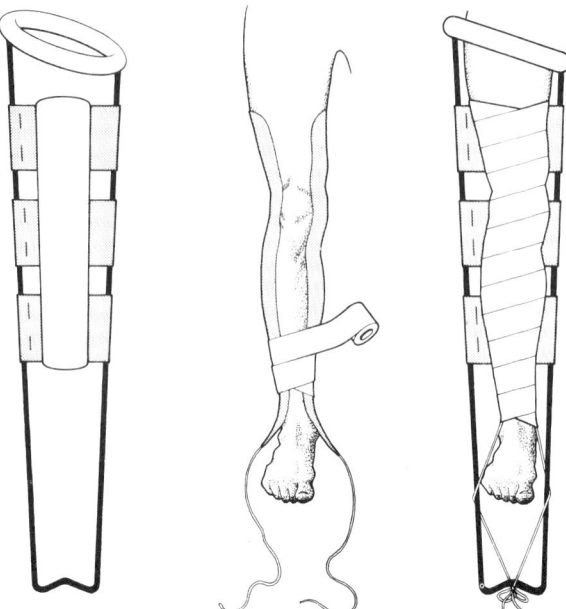

FIG. 26.2. Thomas' splint.

the foot of the bed and inclining the bed head down. This latter method is popular in children's hospitals.

In this fixed traction arrangement the tendency for the limb distal to the fracture to roll outwards is reduced by leading the tapes around the longitudinal struts of the splint before tying them to the cross-piece at the foot of the splint.

The average time taken for union to occur with this method of treatment is 6 weeks in a child and 12–16 weeks in an adult. Most surgeons then advise the use of a caliper to protect the fracture when the patient walks. It is kept on until the fracture has consolidated. During this period attention is directed towards regaining knee flexion.

Other methods of fixation. Although the vast majority of fractures of the femur can be treated by traction, occasionally internal fixation is required. This is achieved either by the use of plates and screws or by the insertion of an intramedullary rod as described by Küntscher.

In children who are too young to allow the use of the Thomas splint, the 'gallows traction' can be used. In this technique adhesive strapping is applied to both lower limbs and the baby nursed with both legs straight up in the air, the tapes being attached to an overhead boom.

Very occasionally a plaster of Paris hip spica may be used to immobilize a fractured femur in a young child.

Complications
1. *Damage to the femoral artery.* This complication is rare. Damage to the artery causes ischaemia of the limb below the level of the injury and loss of the popliteal pulse and the dorsalis pedis and posterior tibial pulses.

If the circulation is not restored by reduction of the fracture, exploration and repair of the artery is necessary. This is usually done with the help of the vascular surgeons. Although the arterial repair is probably better protected if internal fixation of the fracture is carried out, not all fractures require it.

2. *Haemorrhage*. It has been estimated that a simple fracture of the femur causes a drop of between 1 and 2 litres of circulating blood volume. This is due to bleeding and loss of fluid into the surrounding tissues. Although it is not required by all patients, transfusion must be considered and facilities kept available.

3. *Delayed union*. This, as mentioned above, is rare and when it occurs should be treated by internal fixation and onlay grafting. Grafts are usually taken from the iliac crest. Delayed union is commoner in compound fractures.

27 The knee region

ANATOMY

The knee joint actually comprises three joints:
(1) the patello-femoral;
(2) the medial tibio-femoral;
(3) the lateral tibio-femoral.

The patello-femoral joint
This is a sliding joint between the lower end of the femur and the patella—a sesamoid bone enclosed in the quadriceps expansion which, by its position, increases the mechanical efficiency of this muscle in extending the knee.

The tibio-femoral joints
These are gliding joints—the medial having a greater antero-posterior diameter than the lateral. In addition to the hinge action of the knee, some rotation of the femur on the tibia takes place at the end of extension.

Muscles acting on the knee joint
The quadriceps femoris, a four-headed muscle, is the main extensor of the knee—it consists of the vastus medialis, vastus lateralis, vastus intermedius, and rectus femoris. Its insertion into the tibia is by means of the quadriceps expansion—a tough sheet of fibrous tissue which spreads out anteriorly, medially, and laterally around the knee joint and encloses the patella. From the lower pole of the patella, the patellar tendon passes down to the tubercle of the tibia and it is continuous with the quadriceps expansion on either side. This whole system is known as the extensor mechanism of the knee.

There are various other tendons and muscles passing over the knee joint and affecting it. They are:
(1) the medial hamstrings—semimembranosus, semitendinosus, and gracilis;
(2) the lateral hamstrings—biceps;
(3) the sartorius, which passes anterior to the hip joint and posteromedially to the knee.

All these muscles act as flexors of the knee.

In addition, the two heads of gastrocnemius actually pass over the back of the knee joint, as they have a point of origin on the posterior surface of the lower femur. The gastrocnemius therefore acts as a flexor of the knee in addition to its better known function as plantar flexor of the ankle. This action is made use of in some of the operations done for spastics in which the overacting hamstrings are disconnected from the tiba, and re-attached to the femur to act as extensors of the hip.

The patella usually develops from one ossific nucleus but occasionally from two or three. If the areas of ossification do not fuse the condition of bipartite or tripartite patella results. The appearance of this condition on X-ray may be mistaken for a fracture of the patella. It is often bilateral.

CLINICAL CONDITIONS OF THE KNEE REGION

Bursae around the knee joint

Although the anatomists describe sixteen bursae in the region of the knee only three are of clinical significance.

Prepatellar bursitis

The bursa is subcutaneous lying anterior to the patella. Classically it becomes inflamed in patients who habitually kneel forward on their knees, e.g. housemaids who scrub the floors on all fours, hence the popular name for the condition 'housemaid's knee'. Small palpable nodules of fibrous tissue are often found in the bursa.

The bursa may be very swollen and inflamed, in which case aspiration is advised. If the fluid is found to be infected the relevant antibiotic is given. Recurrent attacks of swelling and/or inflammation are best treated by removal of the bursa.

Infrapatellar bursitis

This is a similar condition except that in this case the bursa is lower in position —over either the patellar tendon or the tibia. It is common in people who kneel in the more erect posture, hence the common name 'vicar's knee'.

Semimembranosus bursitis

This bursa lies deep to the tendon of the semimembranosus muscle as it passes over the medial aspect of the back of the knee joint (Fig. 27.1). The bursa tends to swell into the fatty and areolar tissue in the popliteal space, presenting as a fluctuant swelling on the medial side of the space which is not normally tender.

It is seen in two distinct age groups: children and those over 45 years of age. In children the swelling may undergo spontaneous remission and for this reason expectant treatment is often advised. In middle-aged and elderly patients the swelling does not usually subside, and if troublesome, the bursa should be removed. Before excision of the swelling is undertaken, careful examination should be carried out for neurological and vascular changes in the limb distal to the knee because, although rare, neurofibromata and aneurysms of the popliteal artery may also present in this way.

If the bursa has been swollen for a long time it may track down over the posterior surface of the gastrocnemius for some distance and appear as a swelling of the calf rather than the popliteal space.

Recurrence of the cyst is occasionally seen, especially in children.

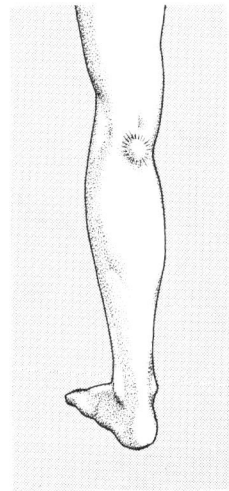

FIG. 27.1. The common site for presentation of semimembranosus bursae.

Baker's cyst

In some cases the swelling is found to communicate with the cavity of the knee joint and if the knee is also affected with degenerative arthrosis, the name Baker's cyst is applied to it.

Chondromalacia patellae

This condition is characterized by degeneration of the hyaline articular cartilage, which lines the back of the patella and articulates with the lower end of the femur. This particular articulation is subjected to great pressure when the patient gets up from the sitting position or takes weight on the flexing or extending knee, e.g. when going up or down stairs. The condition is particularly common in adolescent girls or in young men who subject their knees to great stress, e.g. climbers and soldiers in training.

If one examines the cartilage on the back of the patella in these cases it is found to be shredded and a similar degeneration may be found in the cartilage on the anterior aspect of the lower femur.

Clinical features

The knee may be heard or felt to click on flexion–extension movements and pressing the patella against the femur as the patient contracts the quadriceps may cause discomfort. Comparison with the other knee is often helpful. Differentiation from tears of the medial meniscus may be difficult but it is important to remember that meniscus lesions are relatively rare in young women and common in young men.

Treatment

Resting the knee for several weeks is often all that is required. Very occasionally splinting may be indicated.

Prognosis

In adolescent girls the outlook is good and in most cases the pain settles. In men, however, the prognosis should be guarded as the condition may progress to degenerative arthrosis.

Degenerative arthrosis of the knee

The knee is second only to the hip in importance in osteoarthrosis. Primary osteoarthrosis is common and affects women more commonly than men. The condition is commonest in the patello-femoral articulation, probably because of the enormous pressure that it has to take in such movements as getting up from a chair or climbing stairs. It is also common in the medial femoro-tibial compartment where it is associated with a bow-leg deformity. The question of cause and effect arises here but most patients are adamant that the deformity came on after the pain.

Treatment

This follows the general principles of treatment for osteoarthrosis in other weight-bearing joints, namely weight reduction (diet and walking-stick), warmth, and analgesics. Hydrocortisone injections may help but should be limited to two because of the danger of irreversible damage to bone and articular cartilage.

Failure of conservative treatment is the usual indication for operative measures. These are:

1. Tibial osteotomy, which gives the surgeon the opportunity of correcting any deformity.
2. Arthrodesis, which virtually guarantees pain relief but makes the limb difficult to manage, e.g. on stairs or on the bus, and should be avoided as a bilateral procedure if at all possible.
3. Arthroplasty, which may be either of the tibial condyle replacement type (Macintosh) or the insertion of new bearing surfaces to both femoral and tibial condyles. There are many examples of this type in use and in time we will probably be able to decide which is the most suitable.
4. Patellectomy, which gives good results in cases in which the degeneration is limited to the patello-femoral joint.

Rheumatoid disease

The knee is the commonest of the large joints to be affected by rheumatoid disease. Early symptoms are pain and stiffness, and effusions are commonly seen. As the disease progresses the articular cartilage becomes damaged, with the almost inevitable superimposition of degenerative arthrosis. Wasting of the quadriceps is common. As with all rheumatoid manifestations, sudden resolution may occur for no obvious reason although a gradually progressive course is more common.

Treatment

The general management of the patient with rheumatoid disease is usually carried out by the physician or rheumatologist. The orthopaedic surgeon carries out the local management of the joint.

If the effusions are persistent and large, they are aspirated and the knee is then treated with compression bandaging for 2–3 weeks. If effusions recur for several months or years and are associated with synovial hypertrophy, synovectomy is often advised. This usually cures the condition as far as the knee is concerned, but there is a significant proportion of cases in which the synovium reforms and effusions again occur.

The other operative procedures carried out are really indicated because the condition has progressed to secondary osteoarthrosis. Of the procedures mentioned, arthrodesis is still accompanied by a high success rate and 'total knee replacements' are being used more and more as refinements in technique and implants are made.

Meniscus lesions

The menisci consist of two fibrocartilaginous structures, the shapes of which resemble segments of an orange. They lie on the plateaus of the tibia (medial and lateral) and articulate with the femoral condyles. The medial meniscus is larger than the lateral—as is the corresponding plateau—and its ends tend to enclose the ends of the lateral meniscus. Both menisci are attached by their ends to the tibial crest and by their 'greater curves' to the upper tibia via the coronary ligaments (Fig. 27.2(a)).

Discoid meniscus
On occasion the lateral meniscus, instead of being crescentic in shape is more rounded, appearing as a circular disc and being named a discoid meniscus.

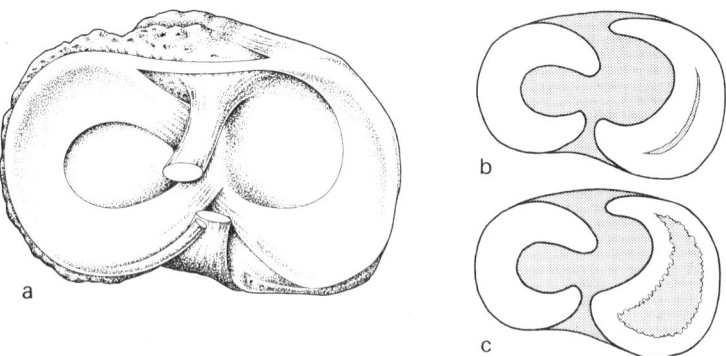

FIG. 27.2. (a) The appearance of the menisci when viewed from above. (b) A longitudinal split of the medial meuiscus. (c) A 'bucket-handle' tear of the medial meniscus.

This may give rise to clicking in early life or discomfort and instability in adult life. Excision is recommended if the symptoms warrant it.

Tears of the menisci
Tears are commoner in the medial than in the lateral meniscus. The mechanism of tearing is usually by sustaining a rotation strain on the weight-bearing flexed knee and, as can easily be appreciated, these lesions are common in sports injuries, especially in football. The common lesions found are longitudinal splits and bucket-handle tears (Fig. 27.2).

The characteristic history is that of a sudden strain to the knee which causes acute pain followed later by swelling and instability. The patient usually seeks medical advice and has the knee immobilized for a period. During the ensuing months the knee tends to buckle or 'give way', particularly when subjected to a twisting strain, and may 'lock' on occasion.

In orthopaedic parlance a specific definition has been given to the word 'lock': by it we mean that the ability to extend the knee fully is lost, but the ability to flex it is retained. This use of the word 'lock' therefore differs from the conventional English usage.

It is equally important to enquire of the patient how he 'unlocks' the joint because we often find that after a few episodes of 'locking' the patient finds finds that he can 'unlock' the joint by some manipulative manoeuvre such as pressing on the medial meniscus or rotating the tibia while not taking weight on the leg.

Recurrent effusion following giving way or locking episodes are common and may lead to stretching of the capsule of the knee joint and subsequent increase in the travel of the tibia in the draw test (p. 11).

Clinical signs
The quadriceps muscle may be wasted—minor degrees of wasting being identified by measuring the girth of the thigh.

The range of movement of the knee may be limited. This applies particularly to extension where the knee movement stops 5–10° short of full and if the examiner gently strains the knee an impression of a rubbery block is obtained, as though a piece of india-rubber has been placed between tibia and femur to stop full extension. This is probably the most dependable sign of a meniscus tear.

There may be an increased travel of the tibia on the draw test, either because of recurrent effusions or because of concomitant damage to the anterior cruciate ligament.

There may be pain or laxity on testing the medial ligament of the knee. Tearing of the medial meniscus, medial ligament, and anterior cruciate ligament are sometimes seen as a characteristic triad of lesions in severe injuries of the knee.

The commonest sign of a meniscus tear is tenderness over the medial joint line—sometimes felt over the anterior end of the meniscus, but more commonly over a point deep to the medial ligament.

McMurray's test (p. 12) may be positive.

Prognosis

It is important to realize that menisci are nourished by the synovial fluid. Having no blood-supply, they are unable to undergo repair by the usual methods and therefore once a meniscus has been torn it remains torn. As far as treatment is concerned therefore there is only one decision to be made—should the meniscus be removed or not? This decision is influenced by two factors: the age of the patient and the severity of the symptoms. If the patient is over, say, 35 years of age it is unlikely that this knee will return to normal after meniscectomy: he may have some instability and swelling from time to time. On the other hand, the young footballer of 18–25 years of age will probably have a normal or near-normal knee after meniscectomy. We would not therefore advise meniscectomy in an older patient with minimal symptoms but would advise it in a younger patient, e.g. a scaffolder whose knee tended to give way and constitute a real danger to him.

Meniscectomy

This is the commonest operation done in most orthopaedic trauma units. The routine in our units is a 2-day pre-operative preparation of the limb (including quadriceps exercises). A standard meniscectomy using the Robert Jones curved incision (following the line of the femoral condyle) is then carried out. Postoperatively the patient spends a week in bed. The knee is immobilized on a back splint and the patient performs quadriceps exercises, both of the 'static bracing' and 'straight leg raising' varieties. At the end of the first postoperative week the patient is allowed up—with crutches if he feels he needs them—and, when walking confidently, he goes home. On the fourteenth postoperative day he returns to have his sutures removed and then attends the physiotherapy department for knee-flexion exercises. He continues to wear his back splint when walking because any sudden flexion may cause the knee to swell. As soon as he can flex the knee to 90° the back splint is discarded and he then wears a supporting crêpe bandage only.

The average young patient can return to work at 4–5 weeks after operation if he has a sedentary job or 7–8 weeks if he has an active job.

Regeneration of menisci

There is no doubt that menisci do regenerate after removal and the regenerated meniscus may itself be torn. An orthopaedic unit in Sheffield have three bottled specimens of torn menisci removed from the same compartment of the same knee of a professional footballer.

Cysts of the menisci

Cyst formation is seen more commonly in the lateral meniscus than in the medial. If the cyst is small it may be totally enclosed in the meniscus, if larger it presses outwards and may be visible and palpable on the outer side of the knee. Characteristically the swelling is tense and hard—therefore diagnosed by the uninitiated as an osteoma—and is situated just below the joint line.

As it is connected to the lateral meniscus it moves with the tibia over the range of flexion of the knee and varies in prominence depending on the position of the knee. It is most prominent at about 60° of flexion and often disappears on full flexion of the knee.

Cysts do occur occasionally in association with the medial meniscus but here tend to be softer and larger.

In most cases these cysts are associated with either tears or degeneration in the meniscus and are treated by excision of both cyst and meniscus. This applies to both medial and lateral meniscus cysts.

Injuries of the extensor mechanism

This subject is more easily understood if one considers the extensor mechanism as a whole and appreciates that the injuries tend to occur at different levels in different age groups.

The extensor mechanism consists of the quadriceps muscle (the four 'heads' being the rectus femoris and the three vasti), the quadriceps expansion, the patella, and the patellar tendon (Fig. 27.3). Sudden unexpected contraction of this mechanism or sudden flexion strains of the knee may result in a break in its continuity.

Rupture of the quadriceps

This is a lesion of active sportsmen usually between the ages of 15 and 30 years. The common muscle to rupture is the rectus femoris and this usually follows a sudden contraction, for example, the batsman who is unexpectedly called to make a quick run. He suffers an acute pain in the front of the thigh followed

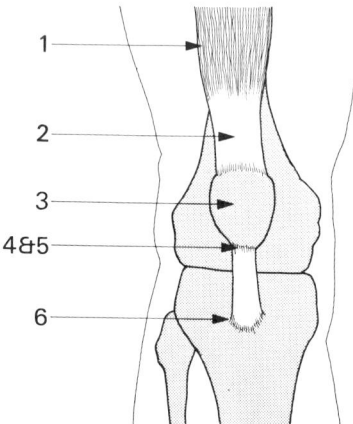

FIG. 27.3. Sites of injury to the extensor mechanism of the knee: (1) quadriceps muscle; (2) quadriceps expansion; (3) patella; (4) and (5) patellar tendon; (6) tibial tubercle.

by swelling over the next few days. When the swelling has subsided, any contraction of the quadriceps causes bunching up of the upper segment of the muscle and a characteristic lump on the anterior aspect of the thigh.

Rupture of the quadriceps expansion
This lesion tends to occur in elderly or the grossly overweight patients. The characteristic story is of a slip going downstairs or stepping onto a nonexistent 'floor' while descending stairs in the dark. Again the symptoms are of pain in lower thigh and, on examination, the patient may be unable to hold the unsupported leg extended.

Palpation reveals a characteristic gap in the quadriceps expansion—sometimes difficult to feel in very obese patients. Treatment is by operative repair.

Fracture of the patella
This is a lesion of middle-age. It must be emphasized that we are describing here the type of fracture due to quadriceps contraction. Other types of fracture of the patella do occur and will be described later.

In this muscle-pull type of fracture the patella separates transversely, usually at about its midpoint. The enormous pull of the quadriceps also causes a tear in the fibrous expansion on either side of the patella; a wide separation of the fragments occurs (see Fig. 27.5). Again the patient is unable to hold the unsupported knee extended, and the position of the fragments may be obvious on palpation.

Treatment consists in operative reconstitution of the extensor mechanism by suturing of the tear in the expansion. The patella may be treated by internal fixation if both fragments are large or by excision of one fragment if it is small —by convention we tend to remove a fragment if it constitutes less than quarter of the height of the patella.

Rupture of the patellar tendon
Complete rupture of the patellar tendon is relatively rare but minor tears are common in young athletes. They tend to occur at the upper end and cause pain on running. If symptoms persist they can usually be successfully treated with a local injection of hydrocortisone.

'Wineglass' avulsion of the patellar tendon
This is a rare lesion but merits inclusion as a connoisseur's item. The patellar tendon is avulsed from the lower pole of the patella, taking with it a part of the periosteum shaped like a bowl. If the lesion is left untreated, this area of periosteum lays down a thin bowl shaped area of bone which on X-ray appears as a 'wineglass' in the region of the upper patellar tendon.

Avulsion of the tibial tubercle
Sudden contraction of the quadriceps expansion may lead to damage to the tibial attachment of the patellar tendon. This is seen particularly in the young in which the 'tongue' epiphysis of the tibia may be pulled upwards. The degree of displacement is usually slight and no treatment is required.

Lesions of the cruciate ligaments
Students sometimes have difficulty in understanding the orientation of the cruciate ligaments. These ligaments are cord-like structures situated in the intercondylar notch of the femur, attaching to the mesial (or opposing) sur-

192 Orthopaedics for Undergraduates

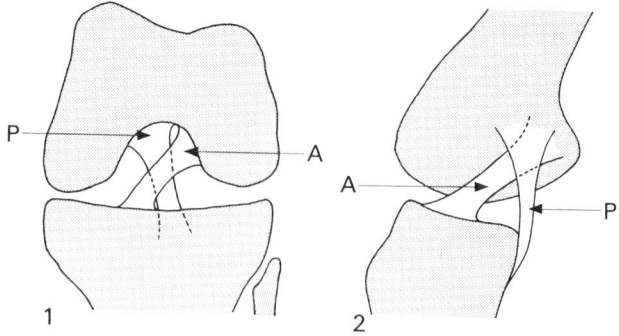

FIG. 27.4. Diagram of the cruciate ligaments. (1) As viewed from the front. (2) As viewed from the side: A, anterior cruciate; P, posterior cruciate.

faces of the femoral condyles and to the crest lying across the upper surface of the tibia in the sagittal plane. They are named from their tibial attachments, the anterior one stretching upwards and backwards from the anterior part of the crest to the inner surface of the lateral femoral condyle and the posterior extending up from the posterior part of the crest to attach to the outer surface of the medial femoral condyle. Since the anterior ligament crosses in front of the posterior one in its upper part they are called cruciate ligaments (Fig. 27.4).

Tears of the posterior cruciate ligament are very rare. Tears of the anterior cruciate ligament do occur and may cause instability of the knee particularly in running. The association of damage to the medial ligament and medial meniscus has already been stressed.

The diagnosis of anterior cruciate ligament tears may be difficult mainly because they are very unlikely to occur in isolation and the instability of the knee due to capsular and collateral (medial or lateral) ligament tears may confuse the picture. For this reason the problem usually presents itself some months after the initial injury and when the patient has returned to full activity. At this stage there may be a marked increase in the draw sign but it must be remembered that previous effusion may have stretched the capsule and this laxity may allow undue movement on the draw test.

Occasionally even examination under anaesthesia may fail to clarify the position and if the instability is a grave disability to the patient operative exploration may be necessary. If the anterior cruciate ligament is found to be torn substitution by gracilis or semitendinosus as a tendon-transfer procedure, described by Lindemann, is carried out.

Lesions of the collateral ligaments

The medial ligament of the knee is a wide structure and tears seldom involve its full width. For this reason operative repair is seldom indicated unless the damage is severe.

The lateral ligament in contrast is a cord-like structure and if torn is unlikely to heal satisfactorily. Operative repair is therefore usually undertaken.

Dislocation of the patella

It should be realized that there is an abuse of teminology here but convention

has justified the use of the above diagnosis rather than the more correct 'dislocation of the patello-femoral joint'.
There are three types of dislocation of the patella:
(1) traumatic dislocation;
(2) recurrent dislocation;
(3) habitual dislocation.

Traumatic dislocation of the patella
In common with other joints the patello-femoral joint may be dislocated in injuries to the knee. Road accidents and sports injuries are the usual causes, and the patella becomes displaced either medially or laterally. Some damage to the capsule is inevitable but repair of the capsule is seldom necessary. Manipulative reduction and immobilization of the knee in extension for 3–4 weeks usually suffices.

Recurrent dislocation of the patella

This is a disabling condition, usually seen in adolescent girls and young adult women. The aetiology is obscure, but two main theories are put forward to explain it: first, that with the widening of the pelvis at puberty, the pull of the quadriceps becomes more obliquely applied to the patella and tends to cause lateral dislocation of it; and secondly that the development of the lower end of the femur is deficient either from the point of view of shape or rotation.

Symptoms. The patient usually states that the knee suddenly buckles for no obvious reason. She falls to the ground and on looking at the knee finds that the patella has dislocated laterally. A word of caution is in order here: with the patella dislocated, the outline of the knee changes and the medial femoral condyle becomes more obvious—some patients think this is the patella and so describe the displacement kneecap as being medial rather than lateral.

Reduction is usually easy but redislocation is common with the result that the patient loses confidence in her knee.

Signs. The knee is usually essentially normal to examination—some authorities have described X-ray evidence of a low profile to the lateral femoral condyle when viewed from above. Others have described the patella as being 'higher', i.e. the patellar tendon is longer than usual. The most dependable sign, however, is what is referred to as a positive 'apprehension test'. This is carried out in two stages. First the patient is persuaded to sit with her legs straight out in front of her and with the quadriceps relaxed. The examiner then gently pushes the kneecap laterally observing the patient's face as he does so. A patient who has a patella which is likely to dislocate immediately registers apprehension as she feels that the patella will pass over the lateral femoral condyle.

If the above test is negative, lateral pressure of the patella is maintained while the patient slowly flexes the knee. In some cases apprehension is experienced in this part of the test rather than in the first part. In some cases the patella does, in fact, dislocate, thus proving the diagnosis.

Treatment. Operative re-fashioning of the front of the knee is carried out. The object of the various described procedures is to tighten up the capsule on the medial side of the knee and loosen it on the lateral side by means of transferring a segment of capsule (Krogius operation), or to move the insertion of the patellar tendon medially and so realign the extensor mechanism (Goldthwait and tibial tubercle transfer). The latter procedure involves an osteotomy of the tibial tubercle and should not be undertaken during the growing period of the tibia because of the danger of premature closure of the growth plate.

Habitual dislocation of the patella
This condition is seen in young children, and the term 'habitual' is used if the patella dislocates every time the knee is flexed. Again, the dislocation is to the lateral side. Sometimes the child is brought to hospital in the pre-dislocating phase because the mother has noticed that knee flexion is limited. If these children are kept under observation many are seen to develop habitual dislocation. Once the patella has started to dislocate the range of flexion increases.

Aetiology. It can be shown at operation that most of these children have a fibrous area in the lateral side of the quadriceps muscle—either vastus lateralis or vastus intermedius or both. The cause of this fibrous area is unknown, but many of these children have a history of injections into the thigh especially in infancy, e.g. for infections or other illness. The fibrous band restricts the travel of the patella and predisposes to its lateral displacement.

Treatment. Operative excision or lengthening of the fibrous band usually cures the condition but may have to be repeated as the child grows.

Fractures in the knee region

Condylar fractures of the femur
These are relatively common in road injuries and may involve one or both condyles. There is also a severe T-shaped fracture of the lower femur which results in both femoral condyles being separated from each other and from the lower end of the shaft of the femur.

Our practice is to treat these fractures conservatively by immobilization by traction on a Thomas splint if an acceptable position can be obtained by manipulation. Open reduction with or without internal fixation may however be required.

Fractures of the patella
The horizontal splitting fracture due to quadriceps pull has already been described. Two other types of fracture of the patella are seen (Fig. 27.5).
1. Isolated segments of the patella may be fractured by direct violence. Each one must be treated on its merits—if the fracture interferes with the integrity of the smooth articular surface of the patella it must be either smoothed off by reduction or removed.
2. The stellate or 'toffee-in-the-paper' type. You will recall from your schooldays that if you wished to share your slab of toffee with your friends you would retain its wrapping and slap it against the wall to shatter it. The paper could then be removed and the 'fragments' of toffee distributed. In the same way the patella is sometimes shattered by direct violence but, being enclosed in the fibrous capsule of the knee joint, the fragments do not separate. These fractures often unite in acceptable position and are therefore treated conservatively. Early knee movement is encouraged. If, however, the posterior

The knee region 195

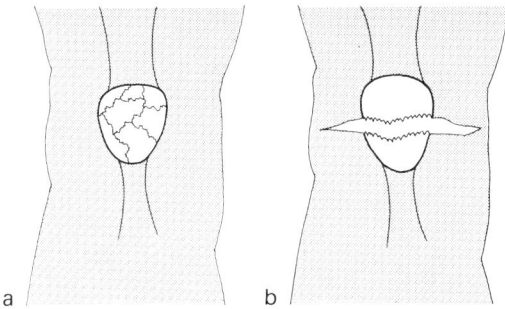

FIG. 27.5. Fractures of the patella. (a) Stellate type—lateral quadriceps expansions intact.(b) Transverse type—lateral quadriceps expansions torn.

surface of the patella has been rendered irregular, excision of the patella is probably indicated.

Excision of the patella causes remarkably little alteration in the appearance of the knee—in fact students are often unable to tell, from a distance, which of the patient's knees has been subjected to patellectomy.

Fractures of the tibial spine
Isolated fractures of the tibial spine are usually due to avulsion caused by straining of the anterior cruciate ligament in hyperextension injuries of the knee. Conservative treatment is usually adequate unless the fragment is considerably elevated from the tibia in which case it can be replaced and fixed in position at operation.

Fractures of the tibial condyles
These fractures, sometimes referred to as plateau fractures, are common in valgus and varus strains and may, in severe cases, cause marked depression of the condyle concerned. If the degree of depression is slight conservative measures are adequate, if severe, open reduction and internal fixation may be necessary. Unfortunately, comminution of the fragments is not unusual and this militates against the success and feasibility of open reduction and internal fixation.

RECOMMENDATIONS FOR FURTHER READING

Du Toit, G. T. (1967) Knee joint cruciate ligament substitution. The Lindemann (Heidelberg) operation. *S. A. J. Surg.* **1**, 25–30.
McMurray, T. P. (1949) Examination of the knee. In *A Practice of Orthopaedic Surgery*, p. 51, Edward Arnold, London.

General references
Smillie, I. S. (1971) *Injuries of the Knee Joint* (4th edn), Churchill–Livingstone, Edinburgh.
Smillie, I. S. (1974) *Diseases of the Knee Joint*, Churchill–Livingstone, Edinburgh.

28 The leg

The following conditions will be discussed:
(1) congenital absence of the fibula;
(2) pseudarthrosis of the tibia;
(3) the anterior tibial syndrome;
(4) fractures of the tibia and fibula.

Congenital absence of the fibula
This is a rare condition but has features in common with the condition of radial club hand.

At birth the child may be noticed to have only three or four toes as the lateral one or two rays of the foot may be absent. Radiographs may show that the fibula is absent.

As the child grows the lateral part of the leg and ankle do not keep pace with the medial and the foot and ankle gradually angle into valgus. Operative exploration reveals that the fibula is represented by a fibrous band.

Treatment
Splintage and periodic manipulation help to keep the deformity to a minimum but operative correction is usually necessary and may have to be repeated as the child grows. Shortening of the leg is common.

Pseudarthrosis of the tibia
This is a rare condition in which the child is born either with a gap in the tibia, usually at the level of the junction of middle and lower thirds, or with a lordotic deformity of the tibia, i.e. the bone is bowed anteriorly. In the latter case the deformity increases as the child grows, and a spontaneous fracture occurs. Non-union is then the rule.

Aetiology
No cause has been found for this condition, and two theories are put forward: (a) that it is a birth fracture occurring at the level of poorest blood-supply in the tibia; and (b) that it is a dysplasia of the periosteum which 'strangles' the bone. The only fact which is known for certain is that some of these patients have neurofibromatosis.

Treatment
Most surgeons use calipers to support the bowed tibia in an attempt to postpone or prevent the fracture of the tibia. Once the fracture has occurred there are two lines of treatment followed.
1. The insertion of an intramedullary pin and onlay bone grafts in the same way as non-union is treated elsewhere. This is not very successful.

2. The insertion of a cortical graft, usually from the other tibia, which bridges the gap and in most cases gradually hypertrophies and takes over the weight-bearing function. This is known as the McFarland bypass graft, after Professor McFarland of Liverpool.

The anterior tibial syndrome

During the Second World War several reports appeared of a clinical syndrome seen in soldiers forced to march for long distances. They developed pain and swelling over the anterior tibial group of muscle which was relieved by resting. If they continued marching, however, the muscles swelled and cut off their own blood-supply. The ischaemia lead to necrosis of this group of muscles. This was known as the anterior tibial syndrome.

It is still seen on occasions but not usually as a fully developed muscle necrosis. It is thought that the fascia which passes from tibia to fibula across these muscles is strong and not distensible and so any rise in pressure within this compartment must imperil the blood-supply.

The syndrome also follows trauma to this area and if a patient develops pain and swelling over the anterior tibial compartment with difficulty in dorsiflexing his toes or foot following a contusion, it is advisable to surgically release the whole anterior compartment of the leg.

Fractures of the tibia and fibula

Although occasionally direct trauma may cause a fracture of one bone of the leg without the other, the majority of injuries cause fractures of both bones. In local practice the majority of fractures of the leg are due to sports injuries and traffic accidents. They are particularly common in motor-cycle accidents, and all patients who have sustained such fractures should be carefully examined for coincident dislocations of the hip. This is especially important to remember when assessing the unconscious patient.

Simple fractures

As in the case of all fractures in the limbs, the initial assessment must include diagnosis of any neurological deficit or vascular impairment in the limb distal to the fracture.

Attention is then turned to the configuration of the fracture line. In fractures due to valgus and varus strains the fracture line tends to be transverse but there may be a triangular fragment of bone, separate from the two main fragments, lying at the level of the fracture. This is called a 'butterfly fragment' (Fig. 28.1).

In fractures due to twisting strains the fracture line will be oblique or spiral in shape.

The transverse type of fracture will be stable to longitudinal compressive forces after reduction but the oblique type, and some of those with a butterfly fragment, will not. This means that, after reduction, the muscles passing over the fracture line will continuously tend to cause telescoping of the tibia. This will result in shortening and deformity of the leg.

This tendency to shortening can be overcome by inserting a Steinmann pin through the lower fragment of the tibia or the calcaneum and incorporating this pin into the full leg plaster cast. A stirrup is attached to the pin and the patient treated in bed with traction applied to the pin. After 4–6 weeks, when

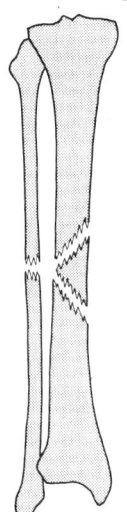

FIG. 28.1.
The 'butterfly' fragment.

union is progressing well, the pin may be removed. It is customary for a test to be done before the pin is removed: a radiograph of the fracture is taken before the traction is discontinued. After 2 days without traction a second radiograph of the fracture is taken. If no significant movement of the fracture has occurred the pin is removed. In some instances two Steinmann pins are used—one through the upper fragment and the other through the lower. They are both incorporated in the plaster.

A transverse fracture with a 'butterfly fragment' which is stable to longitudinal compression can be satisfactorily immobilized in a full-leg plaster cast. The position of the knee is important: it should be held in a position of 20–30° of flexion to prevent rotation at the fracture site. If it is immobilized in the straight position there is a tendency for the plaster to behave like a full-length Wellington boot and, by slipping around the limb, to allow rotation at the fracture site.

Compound fractures

As mentioned in Chapter 3, a compound fracture is a surgical emergency and the connection to the external environment must be closed off as quickly as possible.

The problem with compound fractures of the tibia and fibula is that about one-third of the tibia is covered only by skin and subcutaneous tissue. A large proportion of these fractures are therefore compound and the viability of the skin overlying the fracture is often doubtful.

The most important item in the treatment of the fracture is to achieve viable skin cover. There are many ways of doing this but none is universally successful. Occasionally simple suture of the skin wound, if small, is adequate. Relieving incisions, particularly a vertical one over the calf muscles, may be necessary. The resulting posterior defect is treated by immediate split-skin grafting. Rotation flaps may also be fashioned and the advice of the plastic surgeons is useful in this type of case.

It is our practice to give a course of antibiotics to all compound fractures and, at the time of closure, to remove all necrotic and obviously infected material.

Having ensured adequate skin cover to the fracture, attention is then turned to the fracture itself and treatment carried out along the lines mentioned above. Of course, the opportunity for open reduction is taken at the time of operation but the use of internal fixation is best avoided. If internal fixation is considered necessary it is better to wait 3–4 weeks until the skin has recovered before inserting it. Any shortening of the leg may be prevented in the intervening period by the methods outlined above.

Internal fixation of fractures of the tibia and fibula

Because of its great capacity for uniting, the fibula is seldom treated by internal fixation.

The tibia, however, may require internal fixation and the local practice is to use screws in the long oblique fractures or plates, preferably put on with compression, in other fractures.

Intramedullary fixation is recommended in some centres.

Complications

Neurological complications. Damage to the posterior tibial nerve is surprisingly rare, and in simple fractures should be treated expectantly. In a compound fracture the surgeon may take the opportunity to identify the nerve and, if cut, to mark the ends of the nerve with a black suture. The black suture facilitates identification of the ends of the nerve at the time of secondary suture. Primary suture is only recommended in clean wounds.

The lateral popliteal nerve is more often damaged and the same principles of management apply.

Vascular complications. Damage to the posterior tibial artery does occasionally occur; it may be stretched by the displacement at the fracture site. The first line of treatment is to reduce the fracture. If the circulation does not return after reduction of the fracture, exploration of the artery, preferably with the help of the vascular surgeon, is indicated.

The student should practice and become proficient in identifying the posterior tibial and dorsalis pedis pulses.

Damage to the anterior tibial artery is occasionally seen in high fractures of the tibia. It is very difficult to diagnose but prophylactic incision of the fascial envelope of the anterior tibial compartment should be undertaken in any patient who has swelling in this area with loss of dorsiflexion of the toes and foot.

Arteriography is useful in the investigation of damage to the anterior and posterior tibial arteries.

Compartment syndromes. Swelling and oedema of muscles in the anterior and posterior compartments of the leg may occur in conjunction with fractures. The tense hard swelling and the pain on attempted movement are the indications for operative decompression. Most surgeons take the opportunity to slit these fasciae if they are tight at the time of the operative closure of a compound fracture. If these tense compartments are not decompressed muscle necrosis may result.

Delayed union and non-union. These complications are commoner in the tibia than in most other bones because of the poor vascular supply, particularly to the lower third of the bone. The fibula, being entirely surrounded by muscle throughout most of its length, is very rarely the site of delayed union. Indeed it unites so well that some authorities feel that it contributes to the delayed union of tibial fractures by keeping the fragments apart. Delayed union is particularly likely to occur in double fractures of the tibia; usually one fracture unites and the other shows delayed union.

Treatment is along conventional lines, either by onlay grafting alone or onlay grafting together with internal fixation. Two other lines of treatment are sometimes used:

(a) the use of a 'sliding graft' of normal cortical bone from the tibia above; or
(b) excision of approximately an inch of the fibula to allow better apposition of the fracture surfaces.

The practice of plating the fracture while the fragments are mechanically pressed together (compression plating) appears to have improved the rate of union.

RECOMMENDATIONS FOR FURTHER READING

HARDINGE, K. (1972) Congenital anterior bowing of the tibia—the significance of the different types in relation to pseudarthorosis, *Ann. R. Coll. Surg.* **51**, 17–30.

NICHOLL, E. A. (1964) Fractures of the tibial shaft, *J. Bone Jt Surg.* **46B**, 373–87.

29 The ankle region

ANATOMY

Some aspects of the anatomy of the ankle have important clinical application and deserve emphasis.

1. The ankle is a pure hinge joint between the lower end of the tibia and fibula on one side and the upper articular surface of the talus on the other. The movements of inversion and eversion take place at the joints below and in front of the talus—the sub-talar the mid-tarsal joints.

2. Above the ankle the tibia and fibula are held together by a ligamentous complex which forms a syndesmosis called the inferior tibio-fibular joint. There are three parts to this complex: the anterior tibio-fibular ligament; the interosseus tibio-fibular ligament, and the posterior tibio-fibular ligament. Injuries to the ankle, either of the abduction or the lateral rotation type, may damage two or more of these ligaments.

3. The axis of movement of the ankle joint is at 30° to the coronal plane, i.e. if the tibia is held in the anatomical position, the toes and forefoot move up and down in ankle dorsiflexion and plantar flexion in a line 30° lateral to the antero-posterior plane. This means that if one wishes to obtain a true projection of the ankle mortice on a radiograph the foot must be internally rotated 30° and the rays directed along a line roughly corresponding to the fifth metatarsal.

4. The medial ligament of the ankle is in two parts. The deep fibres are directed horizontally from the medial malleolus to the talus and are therefore very short and thick. The superficial fibres fan out from above downwards and have a long area of attachment to the talus. Their shape accounts for the name—deltoid ligament.

5. The lateral ligament of the ankle consists of three parts:
   (a) the anterior talo-fibular ligament—the most commonly injured part of the ankle;
   (b) the calcaneo-fibular liagment—the most important structure from the point of view of stability of the ankle to inversion strains; and
   (c) the posterior tibio-fibular ligament which is almost horizontal in position and not of great importance in ankle injuries.

CONDITIONS AFFECTING THE ANKLE REGION

For the purposes of description the ankle joint, the sub-talar joint, and the mid-tarsal joint will be considered together.

Congenital club foot

There are three main deformities encountered in the newborn.

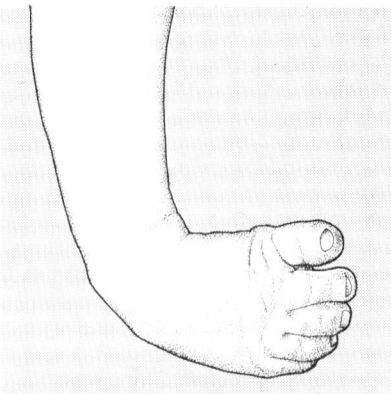

FIG. 29.1. Congenital talipes equinovarus.

(1) congenital talipes equino-varus (CTEV);
(2) congenital talipes calcaneo-valgus (CTCV);
(3) metatarsus varus, which may exist alone or occur as part of CTEV.

Congenital talipes equino-varus (CTEV)
In this deformity, the foot is plantar-flexed at the ankle and inverted (in varus) at the sub-talar and mid-tarsal joints. The heel (calcaneum) is usually underdeveloped and there is often an adduction or varus deformity at the tarsometatarsal joints (Fig. 29.1).

This is the most difficult type of club-foot to treat and constant vigilance during the early years of life is necessary. Treatment is started on the first day of life and is aimed at ensuring that the talo-navicular joint is kept from subluxating and that the tendency to equinus deformity at the ankle is not allowed to develop.

Treatment consists of periodic manipulation of the foot and ankle with splintage during the intervening periods. The varus element of the deformity is corrected first and held by means of a lateral splint. The equinus element is then corrected and the foot splinted in the corrected position. Splintage continues either continuously or for varying periods during the week—depending on response to treatment—until the child begins to walk. This usually occurs at the age of approximately 1 year. Thereafter it may be necessary to alter the footwear slightly to discourage the development of varus, and the child is usually treated in 'night boots' which encourage eversion of the foot and dorsiflexion of the ankle.

Not every case responds satisfactorily to the above routine and more drastic procedures may be necessary: manipulation under general anaesthesia with plaster fixation; and soft tissue operations to correct the deformities, particularly subluxation of the talo-navicular joint.

Occasionally children are seen with established deformity later in life—either because the deformity has relapsed following earlier correction or because it has never been treated. These cases usually require the more severe methods of treatment—moulding and plastering under general anaesthesia, soft tissue correction, and osteotomies of the heel and/or tarsal regions to correct established bony deformity.

The ankle region 203

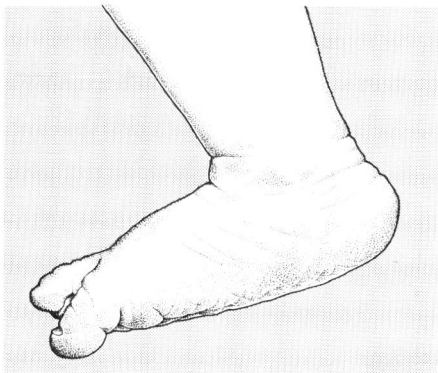

FIG. 29.2. Congenital talipes calcaneovalgus.

Two operations are commonly performed:
1. The calcaneal osteotomy of Dwyer, in which the heel is lengthened and angulated laterally. With subsequent walking the inversion of the forefoot gradually corrects itself.
2. The Dillwyn Evans procedure, in which the talo-navicular joint is reduced by a combination of soft-tissue release on the medial side of the foot and the removal of a wedge of bone from the outer side at the level of the calcaneo-cuboid joint. The tendo-Achilles is lengthened.

Congenital talipes calcaneo-valgus (CTCV)
In this condition the deformity is the direct opposite to that seen in CTEV. Here the ankle is dorsiflexed and the foot everted (Fig. 29.2). There is good evidence to show that the deformity is due to the posture adopted by the foetus *in utero* and treatment by periodic manipulation and application of a splint to hold the foot plantar-flexed is usually all that is required. Relapse is very rare.

Metarsus varus
If occurring on its own in the newborn this condition is treated by manipulation and splintage. Later, alteration to the shoes in the form of an outer wedge to the sole of the shoe (outer flapper) may be advised. If occurring as part of a CTEV deformity, its treatment is included with that of the other deformities. Metatarsus varus is often resistant to treatment but usually improves as the child grows.

INJURIES TO THE ANKLE
Lateral ligament injuries
Sprain of the lateral ligament of the ankle is the commonest sprain encountered in clinical practice. These sprains are usually mild and involve mainly the anterior talo-fibular portion of the ligament. Treatment by strapping the ankle for 2–3 weeks is all that is usually required.

Occasionally the calcaneo-fibular part of the ligament is torn. This injury is caused by an inversion strain and if left untreated will lead to instability of the ankle to inversion strains.

204 Orthopaedics for Undergraduates

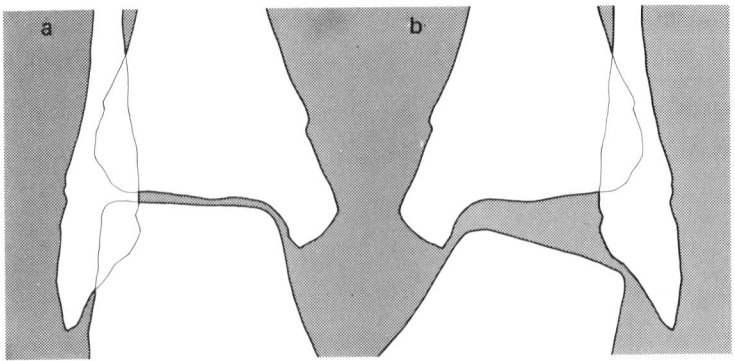

FIG. 29.3. Findings on strain-view radiography of (a) a normal ankle; (b) a tear of the calcaneo-fibular ligament.

The diagnosis may not be apparent when the patient is first seen because of spasm of the peroneal muscles. There will, of course, be tenderness over the ligament, bruising and swelling on the outer side of the ankle, and pain on attempted inversion. In these circumstances the diagnosis is established by strain-view radiography: the patient is given a general anaesthetic and the ankle subjected to a varus strain. A radiograph is taken with the ankle at maximum displacement. If the ligament has been torn an obvious tilt of the talus is seen. The contralateral ankle is also X-rayed under strain for comparison (Fig. 29.3).

Treatment of the complete tear of the calcaneo-fibular ligament is by surgical repair. At operation, the ends of the ligament are found to be shredded and separated. Suturing is difficult but re-alignment of the ends ensures fibrous repair in the most advantageous position.

Chronic weakness of the lateral ligament
This is a common condition resulting in the tendency for the ankle to give way into inversion—referred to as 'going-over' on the ankle. There is usually a history of a previous sprain. Strain-view radiography may show a tilt of the talus.

Treatment of the mild case is by altering the heel of the shoe in such a way that it extends further to the lateral than to the medial side. This has the same effect as an 'outrigger' on a canoe and is referred to as 'floating-out' the heel.

More severely disabled patients require operative treatment of the lateral ligament—usually some form of ligament substitution.

Medial ligament injuries
Because of its triangular or deltoid shape and long area of attachment, the medial ligament of the ankle is not usually completely torn. Separation of the edges does not occur to any significant extent and repair is not usually required. Sprains are less common on the medial than the lateral side of the ankle.

Fractures in the ankle region
Most fractures in the ankle region involve the lower end of the tibia and fibula.

The malleoli—those parts of the tibia and fibula below the inferior articular surface of the tibia—are particularly liable to injury. Fractures usually occur when the position of the foot is fixed by weight bearing and the patient loses his balance. This forces the ankle to bear an unusual strain—a twisting strain or an inversion or eversion strain. The whole of the force is taken on the ankle and fractures and/or ligament injuries occur. Occasionally falls from a height onto the feet cause ankle fractures although fractures of the calcaneum are more common under these circumstances.

In the following descriptions of the mechanism of fractures the term adduction is synonymous with inversion and the term abduction is synonymous with eversion.

Lateral rotation injuries of the ankle
By convention we describe injuries to the ankle as though the foot was moved relative to a fixed tibia—in actual fact, of course, the foot is fixed and the tibia moves, but we use the conventional method of description because the mechanism of injury is easier to picture.

Lateral rotation strains produce the following lesions, the numbers of lesions produced depending on the severity of the injury (Fig. 29.4):
(1) oblique fracture of the lower end of the fibula;
(2) fracture of the medial malleolus or tear of the medial ligament of the ankle;
(3) fracture of the posterior edge of the lower articular surface of the tibia—the so-called 'third malleolus';
(4) a Maissoneuve fracture (see below).

From the list (1)–(3) it can be seen that these injuries may be called uni-, bi-, or trimalleolar fractures.

Treatment. Treatment is by reduction and immobilization in plaster. Reduction is achieved by medially rotating the foot and the plaster cast used to immobilize the fracture must extend above the knee which is immobilized in a position of about 20–30° of flexion. This cast will protect the ankle from being displaced again by a lateral rotation force or other forces.

Open reduction may be indicated if the displacement is not reducible because of soft-tissue interposition (flaps of periosteum in the medial malleolar fracture or dislocation of tendons into the ankle joint). Internal fixation by screws may be required if both the medial and lateral malleoli are fractured in such a manner that the talus cannot be held reduced under the tibia.

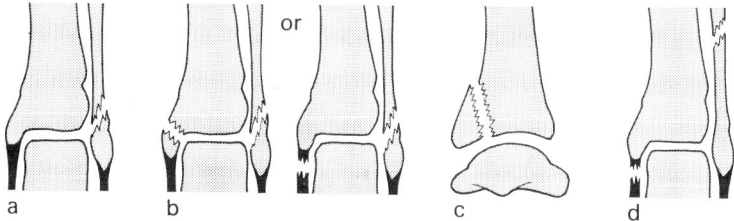

FIG. 29.4. Ankle injuries due to lateral rotation strain. (a) Oblique fracture of the lateral malleolus; (b) fracture of the medial malleolus or tear of the medial ligament; (c) fracture of the posterior malleolus; (d) the Maisonneuve fracture (interosseus ligament tear not shown).

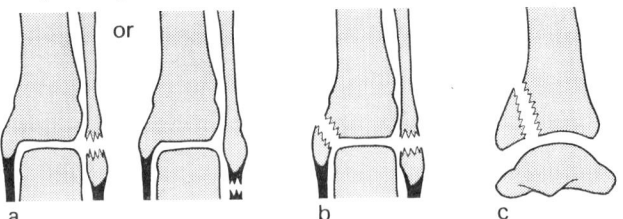

FIG. 29.5. Ankle injuries due to inversion (adduction) strain. (a) Fracture of the lateral malleolus or tear of lateral ligament; (b) 'push-off' fracture of the medial malleolus (c) fracture of the posterior malleolus.

Lateral rotation fractures constitute 80–90 per cent of the ankle fractures seen in our accident departments.

Inversion injuries of the ankle

Inversion strains of the ankle cause the following injuries, the degree of injury again depending on the severity of the force producing it (Fig. 29.5):
 (1) fracture of the lateral malleolus or tear of the lateral ligament of the ankle (see above);
 (2) fracture of the medial malleolus;
 (3) fracture of the tibial malleolus (third malleolus).

Treatment. The same principles apply as to the lateral rotation injuries.

If, on testing the ankle after reduction, it is found that it can be displaced by a lateral rotation strain, immobilization should be in a full 'above-knee' plaster cast with the knee flexed 20–30°.

Eversion injuries of the ankle

Eversion strains will cause the following injuries, the degree depending on the severity of the injury (Fig. 29.6):
 (1) tear of the medial ligament or fracture of the medial malleolus;
 (2) fracture of the lateral malleolus;
 (3) fracture of the 'third malleolus';
 (4) a high fibular fracture (see below).

The same principles of treatment as outlined in the previous section apply for (1)–(3).

Maisonneuve fractures

As mentioned above, a lateral rotation strain may, instead of causing fractures of both malleoli, cause a tear of the anterior and interosseus tibio-fibular

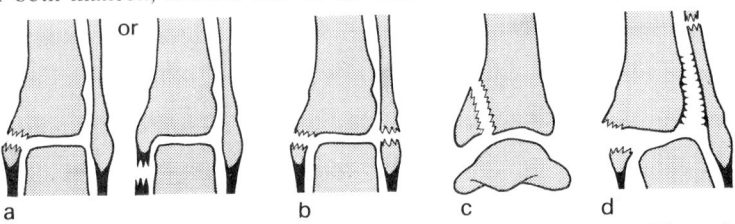

FIG. 29.6. Ankle injuries due to eversion (abduction) strain. (a) Fracture of the medial malleolus or tear of the medial ligament; (b) fracture of the lateral malleolus; (c) fracture of the posterior malleolus; (d) high fracture of the fibula with tearing of the tibio-fibular ligaments.

ligaments, and a fracture—usually oblique—of the fibula above the inferior tibio-fibular joint. Damage to the medial malleolus or medial ligament also occurs. The fibular fracture may be as high as the neck of the fibula.

Strain-view radiography will then show that movement is possible at the inferior tibio-fibular joint. It is important to be aware of these injuries because by the time they are seen in the accident department, the displacement has often been corrected by the first-aid splintage and the diagnosis may be missed.

The combination of a tear of the anterior and the interosseus tibio-fibular ligaments with a fracture of the fibula above the level of these ligaments is called a 'Maisonneuve fracture'.

Treatment. If the medial malleolus is intact, Maisonneuve fractures may be treated by closed manipulation and immobilization in a full-leg plaster cast. In some cases, however, the medial malleolus is fractured in such a manner that the talus cannot be held against it, and it should be fixed in position with a screw. Most surgeons also fix the lower fibula to the tibia with a screw, at the same time. Alternatively, after the medial malleolus has been fixed with a screw the reduction can be held in a full leg plaster cast. The screw across the tibio-fibular joint may require removal after the fracture has united if it interferes with dorsiflexion of the ankle.

High fibular fractures due to abduction

An abduction strain may, on occasion, produce a complete tear of the inferior tibio-fibular ligament complex and a fracture of the fibula above the complex. Damage to the medial malleolus or medial ligament also occurs.

The principles of treatment are the same as for the Maisonneuve fracture: if the medial malleolus is intact the fracture may be immobilized, after manipulative reduction, in a full-leg plaster cast. If the medial malleolus is fractured in such a manner that the talus cannot be held against it it should be fixed in position with a screw. Most surgeons, again, fix the inferior tibio-fibular joint with a screw although it can be satisfactorily immobilized in a full-leg plaster cast.

Vertical compression fractures of the ankles

These are usually severe injuries—often with comminution—and may require internal fixation to preserve the congruence of the ankle joint.

Railing fractures. First described by Professor McMurray in 1931, these fractures were very common in Liverpool at that time. They occur in children and consist of a vertical fracture of the lower tibial epiphysis near its medial end (Fig. 29.7). They are caused usually by the child getting his or her foot stuck between railings and then falling and subjecting the ankle to an inversion strain. Treatment is by reduction and plaster-cast fixation. The important complication of this injury is premature closure of the epiphyseal cartilage at the site of injury with development of a varus deformity in the ankle region as the child grows.

Fracture of the talus. It will be remembered there are no muscles or tendons attached to the talus. It is also unfortunately true that its blood-supply is poor. Fractures through the body or neck of the talus are complicated by a high rate of avascular necrosis of the posterior fragment which becomes distorted and may lead to degenerative arthrosis of the ankle joint.

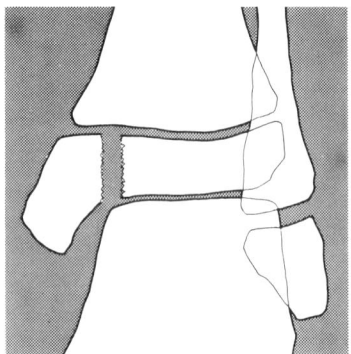

FIG. 29.7. 'Railing' fracture.

Minor fractures of the upper surface of the neck of the talus are common in footballers. They seldom require treatment and do not cause complications.

RECOMMENDATIONS FOR FURTHER READING

DWYER, F. C. (1963) The treatment of relapsed club by the insertion of a wedge into the calcaneum, *J. Bone Jt Surg.* **45B**, 67–75.

EVANS, D. (1961) Relapsed club foot, *J. Bone Jt Surg.* **43B**, 722–33.

FRIPP, A. T. and SHAW, N. E. (1967) *Club Foot*, E. & S. Livingstone, Edinburgh.

30 The foot and toes

ANATOMY

When a person stands, the weight of the body is taken normally on three points of the foot—the posterior part of the os calcis, the head of the first metatarsal, and the head of the fifth metatarsal. These three points constitute a triangle and the weight-bearing line of the limb falls within the triangle. Any deflection of the weight-bearing line outside this triangle will lead to progressive deformity of the foot.

The arches of the foot

The bones of the foot—tarsal and metatarsal—are arranged in a series of arches slung between these three points of weight bearing (Fig. 30.1). There are two longitudinal arches—the medial longitudinal arch between the calcaneum and the head of the first metatarsal consisting of the calcaneum, talus, navicular, inner cuneiform, and first metatarsal, and the lateral longitudinal arch between the calcaneum and the head of the fifth metatarsal comprising the calcaneum, cuboid, and fifth metatarsal. In some people the lateral arch is normally relatively flat.

The transverse arch consists of the heads of the metatarsals and their associated ligaments. This arch often becomes flattened or even reversed

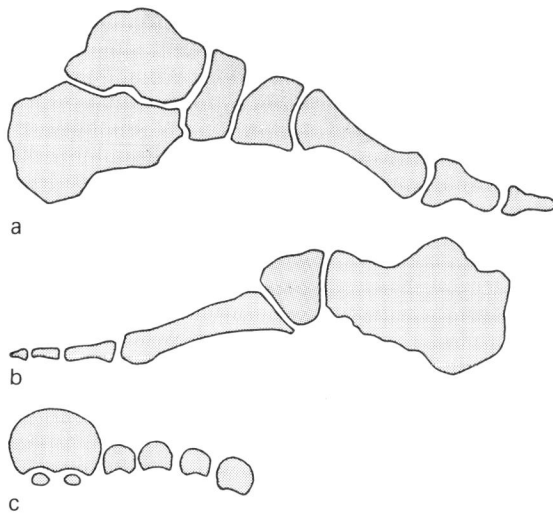

FIG. 30.1. The arches of the foot. (a) Medial. (b) Lateral. (c) Transverse.

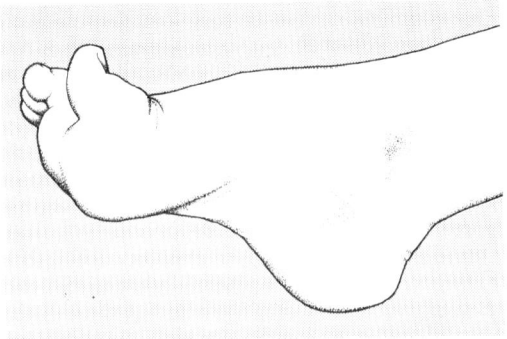

FIG. 30.2. Pes cavus with claw toes.

(convex downwards) in middle age with the production of pain under the heads of the second, third, and fourth metatasals (metatarsalgia).

CLINICAL CONDITIONS OF THE FOOT

Pes cavus

This is a deformity of the foot in which the medial longitudinal arch is more concave than normal. In some cases the calcaneum inclines medially (varus heel) and most cases have some degree of clawing of the toes, i.e. hyperextension of the metatarso-phalangeal joints and flexion of the proximal and distal interphalangeal joints (Fig. 30.2). Symptoms are usually restricted to the toes which develop callosities over the flexed proximal interphalangeal joints. Occasionally callosities develop under the fifth metatarsal base if the patient walks with his foot inverted.

The aetiology of this deformity is obscure but in some cases a definite neurological deficit is demonstrable. This deficit may be associated with spinal abnormalities or a generalized neurological disorder, e.g. Friedreich's ataxia.

Treatment

The clawing of the toes, if severe, is treated by arthrodesis of the interphalangeal joints. The varus and inversion deformity may cause distortion of the foot and require correction which is usually achieved by osteotomy of the calcaneum with insertion of a wedge-shaped bone graft on its medial side (Dwyer osteotomy).

Flat foot

This term is used to describe the deformity of flattening or complete loss of the medial longitudinal arch. It is important to distinguish the congenitally displaced talus (vertical talus) type which is seen in infants, as the treatment thereof is different from that of all other types of flat feet and for this reason it will be described separately later. Peroneal spastic flat foot will also be described on its own.

The other, less severe, types of flat feet tend to be seen at two periods of life:
(1) in growing children;
(2) at middle age.

The foot and toes

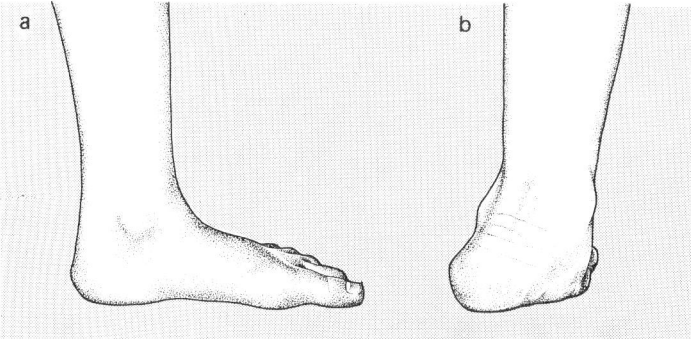

FIG. 30.3. (a) Flat foot. (b) Everted heel.

Flat feet in children
It is very common for children's feet to be flat at some stage during development. Commonly, flattening of the longitudinal arch is associated with valgus deformities of the heels (Fig. 30.3). This implies that the weight-bearing line of the tibia passes medial to the 'triangle' of weight-bearing and that the foot is tending to collapse into valgus. Treatment is by encouraging inversion by means of exercises and by altering the heel of the shoe to tip the calcaneum into slight varus. The inner edge of the heel of the shoe is also lengthened for 1 cm or so to extend the twisting action forward into the region of the inner longitudinal arch. By convention, these altered heels of the shoes are referred to as 'crooked and elongated' heels (C and E heels). These alterations are carried out to all the child's shoes until the tendency to valgus has been corrected and the calcaneum returns to its normal position directly under the tibia. This type of flat foot is often seen in association with a knock-knee deformity.

Grossly valgus feet seen later during the growth period may require surgical correction in the form of osteotomy of the calcaneum.

Flat feet in middle age
The common symptom in association with flattening of the medial longitudinal arch in middle age is aching under the arch—often associated with metatarsalgia. The patients are usually overweight and the pain is due to chronic strain of the ligaments supporting the arches.

Treatment is by physiotherapy (strengthening the muscles which support the arches, both intrinsic and extrinsic), or by the fitting of an arch support—usually fitted to an insole worn in the shoe.

Congenital vertical talus

This condition can often be diagnosed at birth because of the extreme flattening of the longitudinal arch, the loss of plantar flexion and inversion movements, and the prominence of the head of the talus in the sole of the foot.

The condition does not correct with growth and treatment is essential. The basic abnormality is that the head of the talus has lost the support of the anterior end of the calcaneum and has adopted a more vertical position than normal. Consequently it is the neck of the talus rather than the head which

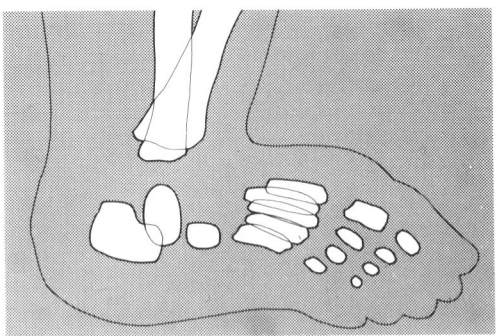

FIG. 30.4. Radiographic appearance of congenital vertical talus.

articulates with the navicula. There is usually some degree of equinus displacement of the calcaneum in addition (Fig. 30.4).

Treatment consists of reduction of the talo-calcaneal and the talo-navicular joints. Opinion is divided as to whether this can best be achieved in one or two stages, but most authorities agree that open reduction of the talo-navicular joint with internal fixation by means of Kirschner wires (steel wire approximately the same gauge as a large sewing needle) is usually necessary. Elongation of the tendo-Achilles may also be necessary.

Peroneal spastic flat foot

This condition is also referred to as 'adolescent spastic flat foot.' Characteristically, the child's foot or feet are symptomless until adolescence and he or she then complains of pain in the ankle area. Examination reveals that the peroneal muscles are in spasm and that sub-talar movement is absent. Any attempt at inversion of the foot causes pain.

Treatment depends on the severity of the symptoms. Mild cases resolve after restriction of activity for a few weeks. More severe cases may require manipulation of the sub-talar joint under anaesthesia.

Very severe cases are best treated by immobilization in a plaster of Paris cast for several weeks.

Radiographs

A large proportion of cases of peroneal spastic flat foot are found to have an abnormal shape of the antero-medial angle of the calcaneum and, if follow-up X-rays are taken, are seen to develop a synostosis between the calcaneum and the navicula (calcaneo-navicular bar). More rarely a bar may develop between the talus and the calcaneum (talo-calcaneal bar). It is believed that the development of these 'bars' is in some way connected with irritation of the sub-talar, mid-tarsal joint complex and that this causes pain and reflex spasm of the peroneal muscles. Some authorities recommend excision of these 'bars' or their precedent cartilage areas in the treatment of the adolescent spastic flat foot.

Plantar fasciitis

The plantar fascia is subject to attacks of inflammation, particularly at its point of attachment to the os calcis. The aetiology is not known but, like inflamed fasciae elsewhere in the body (e.g. tennis elbow), it responds well to the injection of hydrocortisone acetate.

The common physical finding is point tenderness under the calcaneum more to its medial side. The X-ray finding of a calcaneal spur is now thought to be coincidental.

Kohler's disease

This is a relatively common condition in childhood and is an osteochondritis of the navicular bone. Aching in the region of the instep and limping are the main features. There may be tenderness in the area of the navicula and radiographs show density and fragmentation of the navicula. Most cases settle with conservative treatment.

Sever's disease

This is the name given to the condition of osteochondritis of the apophysis (traction epiphysis) of the calcaneum. The child complains of pain in the heel, sometimes radiating up the tendo-Achilles. Differentiation from tenosynovitis of the tendo-Achilles may be difficult.

Radiographs show density and fragmentation of the apophysis, but the significance of this finding is dubious because many asymptomatic heels also show similar radiographic appearances.

Restriction of activity is usually the only treatment required.

Freiberg's disease

This name is given to the condition of osteochondritis of the head epiphyses of the metatarsals. The most commonly affected are those of the second and third toes. The patient complains of pain in the forefoot, there is tenderness to palpation, and radiographs show density and fragmentation of the epiphysis. Symptomatic treatment is usually all that is required.

Often the condition is diagnosed in retrospect when the deformed head of the metatarsal is seen on a forefoot radiograph taken for some other reason.

Hallux valgus

This is probably the commonest deformity seen in orthopaedic clinics. The deformity affects the metatarso-phalangeal joint of the big toe and the phalanges are deviated outwards towards the little toe side of the foot (Fig. 30.5).

As the deformity progresses the metatarsal head becomes more prominent on the medial border of the foot and rubs on the shoe with consequent development of soft-tissue thickening and inflammation, i.e. a bunion.

Hallux valgus is often associated with some varus angulation of the big toe metatarsal so that the forefoot becomes widened—a position aggravated by flattening of the transverse arch. The condition is commonest in middle-aged women who come to the clinic for two main reasons:

(1) the bunion becomes painful; or
(2) the forefoot widening prevents them from wearing shoes comfortably. They spend many hours in shoe shops trying to find shoes which are wide enough and still fashionable.

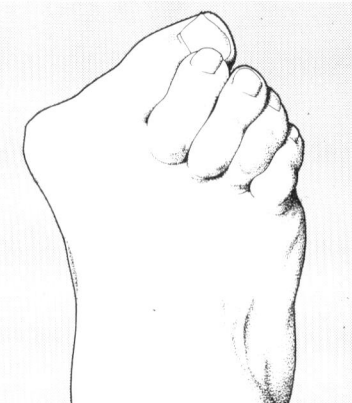

FIG. 30.5. Hallux valgus.

Treatment for hallux valgus in the middle aged is usually surgical. If there is any serious contra-indication to operation, e.g. coronary ischaemia, specially made shoes are prescribed.

The operation commonly used is Keller's operation, which consists of the removal of the prominent part of the first metatarsal head and of the proximal third or half of the proximal phalanx. This leaves the patient with a 'floppy joint' for a few months but with time the ligaments and tendons take up the slack and control of the toe returns.

Hallux valgus is also occasionally seen in adolescents in whom it is usually associated with varus of the first metatarsal. Corrective treatment is seldom indicated but if it is should be confined to an osteotomy of the first metatarsal in preference to Keller's operation.

Hammer toe

This is a deformity most commonly seen in the second toe and often seen in association with hallux valgus. It consists of a position of hyperextension of the metatarso-phalangeal joint, a flexion contracture of the proximal interphalangeal joint and an extension position of the distal interphalangeal joint (Fig. 30.6).

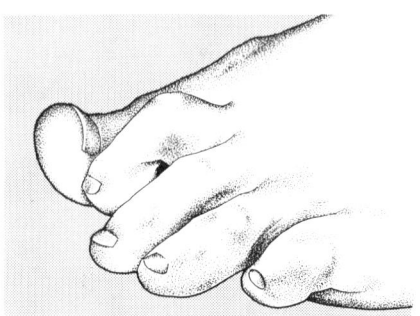

FIG. 30.6. 'Hammer toe' deformity of the second toe.

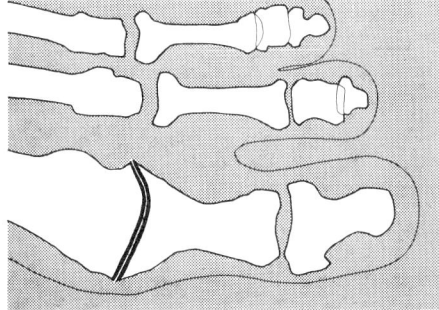

FIG. 30.7. Degenerative arthrosis of the metatarso-phalangeal joint of the big toe: one cause of hallux rigidus.

It should not be confused with a 'claw-toe' in which both the proximal and distal interphalangeal joints are in a position of flexion.

In a hammer toe, symptoms are due to the painful callosity which develops over the dorsal aspect of the proximal interphalangeal joint. The most satisfactory method of treatment is by operative fusion of the proximal interphalangeal joint.

Hallux rigidus

As the name suggests, this condition is characterized by stiffness of the big toe—the joint affected being the metatarso-phalangeal joint (Fig. 30.7). In walking, kneeling, and squatting this joint normally dorsiflexes through a range of approximately 70–80°. Pain and stiffness of this joint interfere with these activities.

The condition is usually seen in patients over the age of 45 years and is due to degenerative arthrosis of this joint. Minor symptoms can be relieved by short-wave diathermy or alterations to the shoes in the form of metatarsal bars and sole stiffeners which produce a 'Dutch clog' effect, encouraging a rolling action of the whole foot in walking and thus diminishing the dorsiflexion strain on the metatarso-phalangeal joint. Patients with more severe symptoms are treated by Keller's operation (see hallux valgus).

Occasionally hallux rigidus is seen in adolescents and young adults. It presents a problem in the athletic type of individual but usually responds to the more conservative methods of treatment. As mentioned in the case of hallux valgus, Keller's operation is not to be recommended in the young.

Claw toes

This condition—a hyperextension deformity of the metatarso-phalangeal joints with flexion deformities of the interphalangeal joints—is seen both in connection with pes cavus and on its own (Fig. 30.8). The aetiology is obscure except in those cases where a neurological deficit or rheumatoid disease is demonstrable. An interesting theory put forward to explain the deformity, especially when occurring in women, is that the custom of wearing tight-fitting shoes leads to lack of movement of the toes, with resultant atrophy of the small muscles of the feet, i.e. the lumbricals and interossei. This has the same effect on the toes as paralysis of the intrinsic hand muscles has on the fingers,

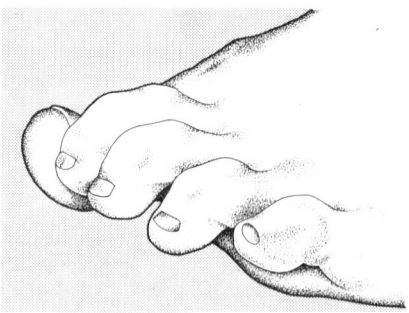

FIG. 30.8. Claw toes.

namely the development of a claw deformity. The foot in this position could be called the 'intrinsic minus' foot.

Treatment is by intrinsic muscle exercises and faradic foot baths in the first instance. More severe cases may require fusion of the proximal interphalangeal joints.

Occasionally the hyperextension deformity of the metatarso-phalangeal joints is so severe that the joints become subluxated or dislocated. If metatarsalgia is marked in these cases, removal of the metatarsal heads and correction of the hyperextension deformity by soft-tissue plication in the sole may be necessary.

Note that in claw toes both the proximal and distal interphalangeal joints are flexed, whereas in hammer toes the proximal interphalangeal joint is flexed but the distal interphalangeal joint is extended.

Ingrowing toe-nails

The tendency for one edge (usually the lateral) of the big toe-nail to grow into the adjacent skin and cause ulceration is usually first seen in adolescence and is referred to as 'ingrowing toe-nail'. Many causes have been suggested but the general feeling is that the condition is idiopathic.

Most commonly the children present with an area of infected granulation tissue along the edge of the nail. Occasionally a less severe case is seen in which the main symptom is pain felt in this area—pain which is aggravated by pressing the skin up against the nail.

Treatment

The less severe cases can be treated by careful cutting of the nail and placing a pledgelet of cotton wool or gauze under the antero-lateral corner of the nail.

Recurrent cases with infection are probably best treated by removal of the nail and the nail bed. The term 'nail bed' is an anatomical one and tends to mislead the patient—nail 'root' is a preferable term for use in discussion.

It is important to ensure complete removal of the nail bed or 'root'—any germinative tissue left will continue to produce small pieces of nail.

Filling the gap resulting from removal of the bed or 'root' sometimes presents a problem because it extends approximately halfway up the distal phalanx.

Two procedures are in common use:

1. Zadik's operation, in which the cuticle is advanced and stitched to the skin which was previously covered by nail.
2. Terminal Symes amputation, in which the distal half of the distal phalanx is excised. This results in more lax tissue being available for filling the defect but, of course, results also in some shortening of the toe.

If the patient presents with an infected ingrowing toe-nail it is customary to advise removal of the nail (under general anaesthesia) followed 6 weeks later by removal of the nail bed or 'root'. The 6-week delay gives time for the infection to settle.

Onychogryphosis

This is the name given to the condition of overgrowth of nails leading, if untreated, to grotesque 'horns'. It is commonest in senile patients.

Most cases can be kept under control by chiropody but occasionally removal of the nail bed or 'root' is indicated.

INJURIES TO THE FOOT

Fractures of the calcaneum

The calcaneum is usually fractured by falls from a height onto the heels and so is common in scaffolders and window cleaners. These fractures are divided into those involving the sub-talar joint complex and those confined to the body of the bone itself (Fig. 30.9).

Those fractures which involve the sub-talar joint usually disrupt its congruence and interfere with the movements of inversion and eversion. The common displacement is impaction of the sub-talar surface of the calcaneum down into the substance of the bone. The normal downward and backward inclination of the bone may also be lost.

Some authorities recommend operative reduction of the sub-talar joint and reconstitution of the normal shape of the calcaneum. This is achieved by inserting a flat bone lever through the posterior surface of the calcaneum, levering up the impacted part of the sub-talar joint and then levering down the posterior part of the calcaneum. The foot is then immobilized in a plaster of Paris cast which incorporates the lever. Three to four weeks later the lever is removed and plaster fixation continued until the fractures have united. The

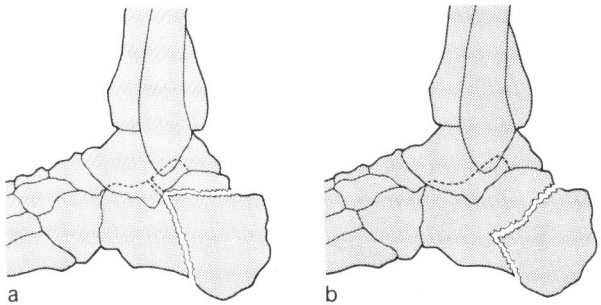

FIG. 30.9. Fractures of the calcaneum. (a) Involving the sub-talar joint; (b) not involving the sub-talar joint.

initial plaster cast immobilizes the foot only but allows sub-talar joint movement, i.e. it is a foot plaster.

Other authorities accept the displacement of the sub-talar joint, apply a wool and crêpe dressing to minimize swelling, and start early mobilization.

All fractures which do not involve the sub-talar joint are treated conservatively in the first instance. Operation may be indicated later to correct painful or troublesome deformities of the calcaneum.

Fracture of the base of the fifth metatarsal (Jones' fracture)

This injury, named after Robert Jones, is of importance in two respects. First, it often occurs in young children, and at this age presents a diagnostic difficulty because there is a separate ossific centre for the base of the fifth metatarsal in this area.

Second, it may signify that a severe inversion injury has been sustained—in which case it may be associated with a tear or sprain of the lateral ligament of the ankle.

Treatment of the fracture is conservative. Mild cases are strapped with protective felt surrounding the base of the fifth metatarsal. Severely painful cases may require immobilization in a below-knee plaster of Paris cast. The coincident lateral ligament injury is treated on its merits (see p. 203).

March fractures

These are stress fractures, i.e. fractures due to repeated stresses rather than a single disruptive force. They occur in the necks of the metatarsals, especially the second, third, and fourth. They derive their name from the frequency of their occurrence in soldiers after route-marches.

These fractures are particularly interesting because they are often difficult to diagnose when the patient is first seen. The break in the bone is often a hairline crack which is not visible on the initial radiograph. Subsequent callus formation makes the fracture more obvious when the X-ray is repeated at 2–3 weeks.

Strapping is usually all that is required to relieve symptoms, although occasionally plaster of Paris casts are used if discomfort is severe.

Fractures of metatarsals and phalanges

These are usually due to direct trauma—especially heavy objects being dropped on the feet. Most fractures are not significantly displaced but occasionally manipulative reduction and, more rarely, open reduction and internal fixation by means of Kirschner wires is indicated.

Compound fractures, especially those of the terminal phalanx of the big toe, may take several months to become symptomless.

RECOMMENDATIONS FOR FURTHER READING

EYRE-BROOK, A. L. (1967) Congenital vertical talus, *J. Bone Jt Surg.* **49B**, 618–27.
RANG, M. (1966) Kellers Operation—original description. In *Anthology of Orthopaedics*, pp. 206–8, E. & S. Livingstone, Edinburgh.
SILK, F. F. and WAINWRIGHT, D. (1967) The recognition and treatment of congenital flat foot in infancy, *J. Bone Jt Surg.* **49B**, 628–33.

Index

abduction fractures of ankle, high fibular, 207
abscess,
  acute osteomyelitis, 41
  Brodie's, 43
  tuberculous, 45
acetabular
  angle, 170
  dysplasia, 170
acetabulum,
  fractures, 177
  Paget's disease, 116
achondroplasia, 58
airway obstruction to, 21
aneurysmal cyst of bone, 80
angle
  of anteversion, 166
  of inclination, 166
ankle,
  anatomy, 201
  dislocations, 204
  examination, 12
  fractures, 204
  osteoarthrosis, 51
ankylosing spondylitis, 109
anterior
  poliomyelitis, 38
    leg inequality in, 39
    scoliosis in, 40
    tendon transfers in, 39
  tibial syndrome, 197
anteversion of femoral neck, 166
apophyses,
  Risser's sign, 103
  Sever's disease, 213
apprehension test, 193
arches of the foot, 209
arterial injuries,
  complicating fractures, 18
  in supracondylar fractures of humerus, 137, 140
arthritis,
  acute septic, 47
  chronic, 48
  in infancy, 171
  osteo, 51; see also arthrosis
  rheumatoid, 33
  Tom Smith's, 171
arthrodoesis, see operations
arthrogryposis multiplex congenita, 85
arthroplasty, see operations

arthrosis,
  carpo-metacarpal joint, 149
  cervical spine, 96
  elbow, 135
  general description, 51
  hip, 51–4, 175
  knee, 186
  operations in, 53
  primary, 51
  secondary, 51
  shoulder, 124
  treatment, 53
ataxia in cerebral palsy, 36
athetosis in cerebral palsy, 36
avascular necrosis
  in cervical fractures, 179
  in Perthes' disease, 172
  of scaphoid, 153
  in slipping of upper femoral epiphysis, 174
  of talus, 207
  in Tom Smith's arthritis, 171
axis, fractures of, 98
axonotmesis, 25

backache, approach to, 106
Baker's cyst, 186
Bence Jones proteose, 79
Bennett's fracture-dislocation, 69, 164
biceps tendon, spontaneous rupture of, 129
bladder, loss of innervation in paraplegia, 112
blue sclera, 55
bone,
  aneurysmal cyst, 80
  brittle bone disease, 55
  diseases of,
    achondroplasia, 58
    chondro-osteodystrophy, 59
    craniocleidodysostosis, 60
    diaphyseal aclasia, 56
    dyschondroplasia, 57
    femoral shortening, 180
    fibrous dysplasia, 66
    hyperparathyroidism, 61
    marble bones, 60
    multiple exostosis, 56
    osteochondrodystrophy, 59
    osteogenesis imperfecta, 55
    osteomalacia, 63

220 Index

bone, diseases of—*contd.*
  osteopetrosis, 60
  osteoporosis, 65
  Paget's, 63
  radius, absence of, 142
  radio-ulnar synostosis, 132
  rickets,
    dietary, 62
    renal, 63
    resistant, 63
  tibia congenital pseudarthrosis, 196
fractures of, *see* fractures
grafts, 199
infections,
  acute, 41
  chronic, 44
  subacute, 43
osteomalacia, 63
osteoporosis, 65
Paget's disease of, 63
tumours of, *see* tumours
Wormian, 55
boutonnière deformity,
  post-traumatic, 162
  in rheumatoid disease, 34
brachial neuralgia, 94
brachial plexus lesions, 26
brittle bones, 55
Brodie's abscess, 43
brown tumours, 61
bunions, 213
bursitis,
  infrapatellar, 185
  olecranon, 135
  prepatellar, 185
  semimembranosus, 185
butterfly fragment, 198
button-hole deformity, *see* boutonnière

calcaneo-navicular bar, 212
calcaneum, *see* os calcis
calcification in supraspinatus tendinitis, 123
calcitonin in Paget's disease, 64
caliper,
  patten-ended, 172
  weight-relieving, 18
callus, 18
cancellous osteoma, 72
capitellum, fractures of, 136
capsulitis of shoulder, 122
carcinoma metastasies in bone, 80
carpal,
  lunate, fracture of, 153
  scaphoid, fractures of, 152
  tunnel syndrome, 30
carpo-metacarpal joints, osteoarthrosis of, 149
carpus,
  anatomy of, 146
  fractures of, 152
cavus foot, 210

central
  cord syndrome, 99
  venous pressure, 24
cerebral palsy,
  ataxia in, 36
  athetosis in, 36
  diagnosis, 36
  operations in, 38
  treatment, 37
  types, 36
cervical
  disc,
    degeneration of, 95
    prolapse of, 96
  fractures (of femur), 179
  neuralgia, 94
  spine,
    anatomy, 91, 97
    dislocations, 98
    examination of, 8
    fractures, 98
    injuries, 97
    intervertebral
      disc-degeneration, 95
      disc-prolapse, 96
    lordosis, 92
    torticollis, 93
    spondylosis, 95
  rib, 96
  vertebrae,
    anatomy of, 91, 97
    fractures of, 98
Charcot's disease, 87
Charnley arthroplasty, 54
chondroma, 75
chondromalacia,
  patellae, 186
  radial head, 134
chondro-osteodystrophy, 59
chondrosarcoma, 76
claw hand,
  total, 156
  ulnar, 27, 157
claw toes, 215
cloacae, 42
club foot, 201
coccydynia, 120
Codman's triangle, 74
Colles' fracture, 149
compact osteoma, 72
condylar fractures,
  femur, 194
  humerus, 138
  tibia, 195
congenital,
  club hand (radial), 142
  definition of term, 3
  hip conditions, 167
  scoliosis, 102
talipes,
  calcaneo-valgus, 203
  equino-varus, 202

Index 221

consolidation of fractures, 16
contracture,
　congenital, of little finger, 157
　Dupuytren's, 158
　Volkmann's, 140
coxa vara, 174
　congenital, 175
　with short femur, 180
　treatment, 175
　types, 175
Craig splint, 168
craniocleidodysostosis, 60
cretinism, 60
cruciate ligament injuries, 191
cubitus
　valgus, 133
　varus, 133
curves of spine, 92

dactylitis, tuberculous, 46
deformity,
　boutonnière, 34
　claw toes, 215
　club foot, 201
　congenital,
　　absence of fibula, 196
　　contracture of little finger, 157
　　talipes,
　　　calcaneo-valgus, 203
　　　equino-varus, 202
　　short femur, 180
　　vertical talus, 211
　coxa vara,
　　causes, 175
　　congenital, 175
　cubitus,
　　valgus, 133
　　varus, 133
　definition of, 3
　dinner-fork, 149
　Dupuytren's contracture, 158
　examination of, 13
　hallux valgus, 213
　hammer toe, 214
　hatchet, of humeral head, 127
　Madelung, 146
　mallet finger, 163
　metatarsus varus, 203
　pes cavus, 210, 215
　radial club hand, 142
　swan-neck, 34
　syndactyly of fingers, 157
　wry-neck, 93
degenerative arthrosis, *see* osteoarthrosis
delayed union of fractures, 19
de Quervain's syndrome, 147
developmental milestones, 36
diaphyseal aclasia, 56
diaphysis, definition, 4
digital nerve, division of, 163
disease,
　Charcot's, 87

　Freiberg's, 213
　Keinbock's, 148
　Kohler's, 213
　marble-bone (osteopetrosis), 60
　Morquio–Brailsford, 59
　mucopolysaccharide, 59
　Ollier's, 57
　Paget's, 63
　Perthes', 171
　Scheuermann's, 101
　Sever's, 213
　Still's, 33
　Von Recklinghausen's,
　　of bone, 61
　　of nerves, 31
dislocation,
　cervical spine, 98
　complications of, 20
　congenital, 132
　definition, 19
　elbow, 139
　finger and thumb joints, 165
　head of radius, 139
　hip, 178
　hip-central, 177
　patella, 192
　　habitual, 194
　　recurrent, 193
　　traumatic, 193
　principles of treatment of, 20
　radio-humeral, 139
　　congenital, 132
　shoulder, 125
　　recurrent, 126
　signs of, 20
　wrist, 154
　　perilunate, 154
　　trans-scaphoid perilunate, 154
drainage,
　in osteomyelitis, 43
　underwater-seal, 22
drop wrist, 27
dumbell tumour of spine, 32
Dupuytren's contracture, 158
dyschondroplasia, 57
dysplasia, acetabular, 170

elbow,
　anatomy, 131
　bursitis (olecranon), 135
　cubitus
　　valgus, 133
　　varus, 133
　examination, 8
　fractures, 136
　golfer's, 135
　loose bodies, 135
　ossification, 131
　radio-humeral dislocation, 132
　tennis, 133
　tuberculosis, 133
elephantiasis neuromatosa, 32

222 Index

endocrine disorders, 60
epiphysis,
  definition, 4
  diseases of, see osteochondritis
  knee, stapling, 40
  slipped upper femoral, 173
equino-varus deformity,
  in cerebral palsy, 37
  congenital, 202
equinus deformity, polio, 38, 39
Erb's palsy, 26
eversion fractures of ankle, 206
Ewing's tumour, 77
exostoses, 72
extensor mechanism of knee, injuries of, 190
fasciectomy in Dupuytren's contracture, 159
fasciotomy in Dupuytren's contracture, 159
femoral
  condyle,
    fractures of, 194
    osteochondritis dissecans, 84
  head,
    avascular necrosis of, see avascular necrosis
    Perthe's disease, 171
  neck,
    angles, 166
    deformity, 175
    fractures, 179
  shaft,
    fractures, 181
femur,
  congenital short, 180
  fractures of, 179, 181
fibroma
  of bone, 75
  of soft tissue, 81
fibrosarcoma,
  of bone, 75
  of soft tissue, 81
fibrous dysplasia of bone, 66
fibula,
  congenital absence, 196
  fractures of, 197, 205–7
fingers,
  anatomy, 155
  deformities, 34, 162
  mallet, 163
  muscle actions, 156
  nerve supply, 156
  stiffness, 165
  tendon injuries, 160
  trigger, 160
flat foot,
  in children, 211
  congenital vertical talus, 211
  in middle age, 211
  peroneal spastic, 212
  types, 210

foot,
  anatomy, 209
  arches of, 209
  cavus, 210
  flat, 210–11
forearm,
  anatomy, 142
  deformities, 142
  ischaemic contractures, 140
fractures,
  acetabulum, 177
  acromion, 124
  ankle,
    abduction, high fibular, 207
    eversion, 206
    inversion, 206
    lateral rotation, 205
    vertical compression, 207
  axis, odontoid process, 98
  Barton's, 151
  calcaneum, 217
  callus, definition, 18
  cervical spine, wedge, 98
  classification of, 15
  closed, definition, 5
  Colles', 149
  comminuted, definition, 15
  complicated, definition, 15
  complications of, 18
  compound, definition, 5, 15
  definition, 5, 15
  femur,
    cervical, 179
    condylar, 194
    neck, in children, 179
    shaft, 181
    trochanteric, 178
  footballer's, 208
  Galeazzi, 144
  greenstick, definition, 15
  healing, complications of, 19
  humerus,
    capitellum, 136
    greater tuberosity, 124
    lateral epicondyle, 136
    lower end,
      comminuted, 138
      Y-shaped, 138
    medial epicondyle, 137
    shaft, 129
    supra-condylar, 137
    surgical neck, 124
  immobilization of, 17
  Jones' metatarsal, 218
  lunate, 153
  Maisonneuve, 206
  mal-union of, 19
  march, 218
  metacarpal, 164
  metatarsal, fifth, base of, 218
  metatarsals and phalanges, 218
  Monteggia, 143

fractures—*contd.*
  non-union, 19
  odontoid process, 98
  olecranon process, 138
  open, definition, 5
  os calcis, 213
  patella, 191, 194
  pathological, definition, 15
  pelvis, 117
  phalanges of fingers, 165
  protection, methods of, 17
  radius,
    head, 139
    lower epiphyseal fracture-separation, 149
    neck, 139
    shaft, 143
    styloid process, 152
    and ulna,
      greenstick, 143
      lower third in children, 145
      shaft, 143
  railing, 207
  reduction, methods of, 16
  repair, stages of, 18
  Robert Jones, 218
  sacrum, 120
  scaphoid, 152
  signs of, 15
  simple, definition, 5, 15
  Smiths, 150
  spine,
    cervical, 98
    lumbar, 110
  stress, definition, 15
  symptoms, 15
  talus, 207
  tibia,
    condyle, 195
    shaft, 197
    spine, 195
  treatment, principles of, 16
  ulna,
    coronoid process, 139
    olecranon process, 138
    shaft, 143
    styloid process, 149
  union,
    assessment of, 17
    delayed, 19
  vertebra, 98; *see also* fracture-dislocations
    lumbar, 110
    transverse process, 110
  wedge, of cervical spine, 98
fracture-dislocations
  ankle, 205
  Bennett, 164
  cervical spine, 98
  Galeazzi, 144
  hip, 177
  Monteggia, 143
  shoulder, 124
  thoraco-lumbar spine, 111
  wrist, 154
fracture-separation of epiphysis,
  radius, 149
  shoulder, 124
fragilitas ossium, 55
Frieberg's disease, 213
Friedreich's ataxia, 210
frozen shoulder, 122

gait,
  antalgic, 13
  athetoid, 13
  drop-foot, 13
  hemiplegic, 13
  rolling sailor, 11
  scissor, 13
  Trendelenberg, 11, 13
  types, 13
Galeazzi fracture-dislocation, 144
ganglia, 69
genu,
  valgum, 3
  varum, 3
Girdlestone's operation on hip, 177
Goldthwait support, 107
golfer's elbow, 135
gout, 83
grafts,
  bone, 199
  tendon, 161
great trochanter, tuberculosis, 44
greater tuberosity, fractures, 124

hallux,
  arthroplasty (Keller's), 214
  fractures, 218
  rigidis, 215
  valgus. 213
hammer toe, 214
hand,
  anatomy, 155
  carpal tunnel syndrome, 30
  contracture of fifth finger, 157
  dactylitis, 46
  deformities, 27, 34, 156, 157, 162
  Dupuytren's contracture, 158
  fractures, 152, 164, 165
  gout, 83
  multiple chondromas, 75
  neurological deformities, 27, 37, 156, 157
  rheumatoid disease, 34
  stenosing tenosynovitis, 69
  tendon injuries, 160
  tenosynovitis,
    acute, 67
    chronic, 69
    subacute, 68
'hanging arm' reduction of dislocated shoulder, 126
Harrison's sulcus, 62

224 Index

heel,
  fasciitis, 212
  osteochondiitis (Sever's disease), 213
Hilton's dictum, 95
hip,
  anatomy, 166
  arthroplasty, 54, 177
  clicking, 168
  clunking, 167
  congenitally dislocatable, 167
  coxa vara, 174
  development, 166
  dislocation,
    congenital, 167
    traumatic, 178
  examination, 9
  fractures,
    acetubular, 177
    femur,
      cervical, 179
      trochanteric, 178
  osteoarthritis, 175
  osteotomy,
    femoral, 54, 177
    pelvic, 171
  Perthes' disease, 171
  slipped upper femoral epiphysis, 173
humerus,
  capitellum, 136
  greater tuberosity, 124
  lateral epicondyle, 136
  medial epicondyle, 137
  ossification of lower end, 131
  shaft, 129
  supracondylar, 137
  Y-shaped, 138
hydrocortisone,
  in golfer's elbow, 135
  in osteoarthrosis, 186
  in tennis elbow, 134
  in tenosynovitis, 147
hyperparathyroidism, 61
hypothyroidism, 60

idiopathic scoliosis, 102
inclination, angle of, 166
infantile
  scoliosis, 102
  torticollis, 94
infections
  of bone, 41
  of joints, 47
inferior tibio-fibular ligament, anatomy, 201
ingrown toenail, 216
internal fixation, 17
  indications for, 17; *see also* individual fractures
interosseus muscle wasting in ulnar palsy, 29
intervertebral disc,
  anatomy, 92

degeneration,
  cervical, 95
  lumbar, 108
prolapse,
  cervical, 96
  lumbar, 106
intrinsic muscles
  of foot, 215
  of hand, 156
inversion fractures of ankle, 206
involucrum, 42
irritable hip, 173
ischaemic contracture
  of calf, 199
  of forearm, 140
ivory osteomas, 72

joints,
  anatomy, *see* individual joints
  degeneration, 51
  diseases,
    arthrogryposis multiplex congenita, 85
    Charcot's, 87
    gout, 83
    infections,
      acute, 47
      chronic, 48
      tuberculous, 48
    osteoarthrosis, general 51; *see also* individual joints
    osteochondritis dissecans, 84
    rheumatoid, 33
    synovial chondromatosis, 78
    synovitis,
      non-specific, 11
      rheumatoid, 33
      transient, of hip, 173
      villonodular, 86
  dislocations, 19
  effusions, 11
  examination, 7; *see also* individual joints
  injuries, *see* individual joints
  loose bodies in, 86
  luxations, 20
  ranges of movement, 8–13
  space, radiological, 8
  subluxations, 20
  villonodular synovitis, 86

Keller's operation, 214
Keinbock's disease, 148
Klippel–Feil syndrome, 93
Klumpke's paralysis, 26
knee,
  anatomy, 184
  bursae around, 185
  Charcot's disease, 87
  effusions, 11
  examination, 11
  extensor mechanism injuries, 190
  fractures, 194

knee—contd.
  genu
    valgum, 3
    varum, 3
  ligament injuries,
    collateral, 192
    cruciate, 191
  locking of knee, 188
  meniscus,
    anatomy, 187
    cysts, 190
    discoid, 187
    tears, 188
  osteoarthrosis, 186
  osteochondritis dissecans, 84
  rheumatoid disease of, 187
Kohler's disease, 213
Krogius operation, 193
Küntscher nail, 182
kyphosis,
  adolescent, 101
  normal, 92
  senile, 65

laminectomy, 108
lateral
  cutaneous nerve compression, 31
  rotation fractures of ankle, 205
leg
  length inequality, 39
    in polio, 39
    true and apparent, 10
  lengthening, 39
  shortening, 39
leukaemia, 79
ligament,
  inferior tibio-fibular, anatomy, 201
  injuries,
    ankle, 203, 204
    cruciate, 191
    knee, 191, 192
    inferior tibio-fibular,
      anterior, 206
      total, 207
    metacarpo-phalangeal joints, 165
    wrist, 149
line,
  Shenton's, 169
  Von Rosen's, 169
locking of knee, 188
loose bodies, 86
  causes, 86
lumbar
  disc prolapse, 106
  spine,
    anatomy, 105
    anomalies, 105
    examination, 9
    fracture-dislocations, 111
    fractures of transverse process, 110
    infections, 105
    scoliosis, 103

spondylolisthesis, 114
spondylolysis, 113
spondylosis, 108
wedge fractures, 110

Madelung's deformity, 146
mallet finger, 163
mal-union of fractures, 19
marble bones, 60
march fractures, 218
M-band in plasma proteins, 79
McMurray's osteotomy, 54, 117
McMurray's test, 189
medial cord lesion, 26
median nerve,
  compression,
    at elbow, 137
    at wrist, 30
  injuries, 28
meningocoele, 105
meniscus,
  anatomy, 187
  cysts, 190
  discoid, 187
  regeneration, 189
  tears, 188
meralgia paraesthetica, 31
metacarpals, fractures, 164
metacarpo-phalangeal joints,
  dislocations, 165
  ligaments,
    anatomy, 159
    injuries, 165
  movements, 155
  muscles acting on, 156
metaphysis, definition, 5
metatarsalgia, 210
metatarsals,
  fractures, 218
  Jones' fracture, 218
  osteochondritis, 213
metatarso-phalangeal joint, examination, 13
mid-tarsal joint, examination, 12
milestones, developmental, 36
Milwaukee brace, 104
monostatic fibrous dysplasia, 66
Monteggia fracture-dislocation, 143
Morquio–Brailsford disease, 59
multiple
  chondromata, 57
  exostoses, 56
  myeloma, 78
muscle wasting, in nerve lesions, 38
musculo-spiral nerve, 27
myelography in disc lesions, 108
myeloma, 78
myelomeningocoele, 105
myositis ossificans, 139
myxoedema, 60

navicular, osteochondritis of, 213

neck,
  cervical,
    neuralgia, 94
    spondylosis, 95
  torticollis,
    infantile, 94
    scoliotic, 94
    spasmodic, 93
  wry-neck, 93
nerve(s),
  examination, 13
  lesions,
    classifications, 25
    complicating fractures, 15, 130
    diagnosis, 25
    division of digital nerve, 163
    electrical tests, 26
    repair, 29
    signs, 25
    treatment, 29
neuralgia,
  brachial, 94
  cervical, 94
  sciatic, 106
neurapraxia, 25
neuritis, ulnar, 29
neurofibromatosis,
  general, 31
  and pseudarthrosis of tibia, 196
  and scoliosis, 32
neurogenic shock, 23
neuroma, 31
neuropathic joints, 87
neurotmesis, 25
non-union of fractures, 19
nucleus pulposis, 106

obturator neurectomy, 38
odontoid process, fractures, 98
olecranon
  bursitis, 135
  process, fractures, 138
oligaemic shock, 22, 23
Ollier's disease, 57
onychogryposis, 217
operations,
  adductor tenotomy, 38
  arthrodesis in rheumatoid disease, 35
  arthroplasty,
    Charnley, 54
    in degenerative arthrosis, 53
    Girdlestone, 177
    Macintosh, 187
    McKee-Farrar, 54
    Moore, 177
    in rheumatoid disease, 35
    Ring, 54
    Thompson,
    Bankart, 128
    Chiari, 171
    in degenerative arthrosis, 53

Dillwyn Evans, 203
  for relapsed club foot, 203
Dwyer, for pes cavus, 210
Eggers, 38
elongation of tendo-Achilles, 38
epiphyseal arrest in long bones, 40
fasciectomy, 159
fasiotomy, 159
femoral lengthening, 39
fenestration, 108
Goldthwait, 194
grafting of tibial fractures, 199
hamstring tenotomy, 38
Keller's, 214
Krogius, 193
laminectomy, 108
Lindemann, 192
McFarland bypass graft, 197
obturator neurectomy, 38
osteotomy,
  in degenerative arthrosis, 53, 187
  McMurray, 54, 177
  tibial, 187
patellectomy, 187, 194, 195
in poliomyelitis,
Putti-Platt, 128
in rheumatoid disease, 35
Salter, 171
Smith-Petersen, 177
Symes terminal toe, 217
synovectomy in rheumatoid disease, 35
tendon transplants in polio, 39
tibial
  lengthening, 39
  tubercle transfer, 194
Zadik's, 217
os calcis,
  apophysitis, 213
  fractures, 213
  osteotomy, 203, 210
  spur, 213
osteitis,
  condensans ilii, 117
  deformans, 63
  fibrosa cystica, 61
  pubis, 117
osteo-arthrosis,
  carpo-metacarpal joint, 149
  causes, 51
  cervical spine, 96
  elbow, 135
  hip, 175
  knee, 186
  primary, 51
  secondary, 51
  shoulder, 124
  signs, 52
  symptoms, 51
  thumb, 149
  treatment, 53
  X-ray findings, 52

osteochondritis,
  dissecans,
    ankle, 84
    elbow, 84, 135
    knee, 84
    heel, 213
    hip, 171
    lunate, 148
    metatarsal head, 213
    navicular, 213
    thoracic spine, 101
osteochondrodystrophy, 59
osteochondroma, 72
osteogenesis imperfecta, 55
osteoid osteoma, 79
osteomalacia, 63
osteomyelitis,
  acute, 41
  bone-scanning, 42
  brucella, 44
  chronic, 44
  of pelvis, 116
  subacute, 43
  tuberculous, 44
  typhoid, 44
osteopetrosis, 60
osteoporosis,
  localized, 65
  generalized, 65
  pathological fractures, 65
  senile, 65
  spine, 65
osteosarcoma, 73
osteotomy,
  femoral,
    in congenital dislocation of hip, 170
    in coxa vara, 175
    in osteoarthrosis, 53, 187
    in Perthes' disease, 172
    in slipped upper femoral epiphysis, 174
  foot, 202
  McMurray, 54, 177
  metatarsal, 214
  pelvic, 171
  spine, 110
  tibial, 187

Paget's disease,
  coxa vara in, 175
  general description, 63
  sarcoma in, 64
pain,
  investigation of, 6
  referred, 95
painful arc syndrome, 123
palsy, see paralysis
paradox, ulnar, 28
paradoxical respiration, 21
paralysis,
  brachial plexus, 26
  Erb's, 26
  facial, 26

  in fractures of humerus, 130
  Klumpke's, 26
  lateral popliteal nerve, 28
  median nerve, 28
  radial nerve, 27
  sciatic nerve, 28
  ulnar nerve, 27
paralytic scoliosis, 101
paraplegia,
  Pott's, 45
  in scoliosis, 103
  traumatic, 111
  treatment, 112
paravertebral abscess, 45
pars interarticularis, 93
patella,
  chondromalacia, 186
  dislocation, 192
    habitual, 194
    recurrent, 193
    traumatic, 193
  fractures, 191, 194
  tap, 11
patellar tendon avulsion, 191
patellectomy, 187, 194, 195
patello-femoral osteoarthrosis, 186
pathological fractures, 15, 64, 65
pelvis,
  acute osteomyelitis, of, 116
  fractures, of, 117
  oystering of, 119
  Paget's disease of, 116
  tuberculosis of, 116
perilunate dislocation of wrist, 154
periosteal fibrosarcoma, 75
peripheral nerve injuries,
  brachial plexus lesions, 26
  Erb's palsy, 26
  Klumpke's paralysis, 26
  medial cord syndrome, 26
  median nerve, 28
  radial nerve, 27
  sciatic nerve, 28
  ulnar nerve, 27
peroneal spastic flat foot, 212
Perthes' disease, 171
pes
  cavus, 210, 215
  planus, see flat foot
plantar fasciitis, 212
plasmacytoma, 78
plexiform neurofibromatosis, 31
pneumothorax tension, 22
poliomyelitis, 38
polyostotic fibrous dysplasia, 66
postural scoliosis, 103
Pott's fracture, see ankle fractures
Pott's paraplegia, 45
profundus tendon injury, 160, 161
prolapsed disc,
  cervical, 96
  lumbar, 106

Putti-Platt operation, 128
pyogenic infection
  of bone, 41
  of joint, 47

quadriceps
  expansion, rupture of, 191
  muscle,
    rupture, 190
    wasting, 188
    weakness, 38

radial
  head
    dislocation,
      congenital, 132
      traumatic, 139
    fractures, 139
  nerve,
    injury, 27, 130
  styloid
    excision, 153
    fracture, 152
radio-carpal joint, dislocation, 154
radio-ulnar synostosis, 132
radius,
  congenital absence, 142
  fractures,
    head, 139
    lower end, 149, 150, 151
    neck, 139
    shaft, 143
    styloid process, 152
reduction of fractures, 16
referred pain, 95
renal
  osteodystrophy, 63
  rickets, 63
resistant rickets, 63
respiration, paradoxical, 21
rhesus incompatibility and cerebral palsy, 36
rheumatoid
  disease,
    hand deformities, 34
    pathology, 33
    signs, 34
    treatment, 35
  factor, 35
rickets,
  deformities, 175
  dietary, 62
  Harrison's sulcus in, 62
  renal, 63
  resistant, 63
rickety rosary, 62
Risser's sign, 103
Robert Jones,
  fracture, 218
  incision, 189
rupture of rectus femoris, 180

sacro-iliac joint,
  radiographic appearance, 116
sacrum,
  fractures of, 120
sarcoma,
  osteosarcoma, 73
  Paget's, 74
  primary, 73
  secondary, 74
scalene muscles in thoracic outlet syndrome 96
scaphoid bone,
  avascular necrosis, 153
  blood-supply, 153
  fractures, 152
scapula,
  undescended, 121
Scheuermann's disease, 101
sciatic nerve injury, 28
sciatica, 106
scoliosis,
  classifications, 102
  effects of, 103
  measurement, 103
  in poliomyelitis, 40
  prognosis, 102
  signs, 102
  symptoms, 102
  treatment, 103
secondary
  osteoarthrosis, 51
  osteosarcoma, 74
  tumours, 80
senile osteoporosis, 65
septicaemia
  in osteomyelitis, 42
  in septic arthritis, 47
sequestrum, 42
serum uric acid, 83
Sever's disease, 213
shelf operation in congenital hip disease, 171
Shenton's line, 169
shock,
  causes of, 22
  prevention and treatment, 23
shortening of leg, true and apparent, 10
shoulder,
  anatomy, 121
  arthrodoesis, 27
  capsulitis, 122
  dislocation,
    traumatic, 125
    recurrent, 126
  examination, 8
  fractures, 124
  frozen, 122
  osteoarthrosis, 124
  painful arc syndrome, 123
  rotator cuff lesion, 123
  Sprengel's, 121
  supraspinatus tendinitis, 123

Index 229

sign,
  Froment's, 28
  MacNab's, 108
  Risser's, 103
  Trendelenburg's,
    in congenitally dislocatable hip, 170
    description, 10
    in osteoarthrosis, 176
sinus formation, in tuberculosis, 49
skull
  enlargement, in Paget's disease, 64
  radiographs in multiple myelomatosis, 79
slipping of the upper femoral epiphysis, 173
Smith–Petersen operation, 177
solitary myeloma, 78
spasmodic torticollis, 93
spastic flat foot (adolescent), 212
spina bifida, 105
spinal
  cord,
    anatomy, 97, 99
    injuries, 97, 99
  fusion,
    in scoliosis, 104
    in spondylolisthesis, 114
spine,
  anatomy, 91, 97
  congenital anomalies, 93, 105
  deformities, 93, 101
  dislocations (cervical), 98
  examination, 8, 9
  fractures, 98, 110
  fracture-dislocations, 111
  intervertebral disc lesions,
    cervical, 95, 96
    lumbar, 106, 108
  kyphosis, 92
  lordosis, 92
  osteoarthrosis, of, 92
  scoliosis, 101
  spondylitis, 93, 109
  spondylolisthesis, 93, 114
  spondylolysis, 93, 113
  spondylosis, 92
    cervical, 95
    lumbar, 108
  tuberculosis, 44
splint
  Thomas', 181
  Craig, 168
spondylitis, 109
  definition, 93
  description, 109
spondylogram, 110
spondylolisthesis,
  definition, 93
  description, 114
spondylolysis, 93, 113
  definition, 93
  description, 113

spondylosis, 92
  cervical, 95
  lumbar, 108
sprains,
  ankle ligaments, 203, 204
  finger ligaments, 165
  knee ligaments,
    collateral, 192
    cruciate, 191
  wrist ligaments, 149
Sprengel shoulder, 121
stenosing tenosynovitis, 68, 69, 147
sternomastoid 'tumour', 94
Still's disease, 33
stove-in pelvis, 177
stress fractures,
  definition, 15
  metatarsals, 218
  in Paget's disease, 64
structural scoliosis, 103
sublimis tendon injury, 160, 161
subluxation, definition, 19
sub-talar joint,
  in adolescent spastic flat foot, 212
  in congenital talipes equinovarus, 202
  in congenital vertical talus, 212
  examination, 12
  in fractures of the os calcis, 217
subtrochanteric osteotomy, 54, 117
supracondylar fracture of humerus, 137
supraspinatus tendinitis, 123
Syme's terminal amputation, 217
syndrome,
  anterior tibial, 197
  carpal tunnel, 30
  central cord, 99
  compartment, in tibial fractures, 199
  Cushing's, osteoporosis in, 65
  de Quervain's, 147
  Felty's, 33
  Klippel–Feil, 93
  painful arc, 123
  radial tunnel, 134
  tarsal tunnel, 31
  thoracic outlet, 96
  ulnar tunnel, 29
synovial
  effusion, 11
  chondromatosis, 87
  osteochondromatosis, 87
synovitis,
  acute, 188
  transient, 173
  traumatic, 188
  tuberculous, 49
syringomyelia, 87

talipes,
  calcaneo-valgus, 203
  equino-varus, 201–2
  talo-calcaneal bar, 212

talus,
   avascular necrosis, 207
   congenital vertical, 211
   fractures, 207
   footballer's, 208
   tears of adductor origin, 117
   technique, hanging arm, for dislocation of shoulder, 126
tendinitis,
   supraspinatus, 123
   tendo-Achilles, 68, 213
tendo-Achilles,
   elongation of, 38
   inflammation of, 68, 213
   rupture, 69
   tightness, in club foot, 202
      in cerebral palsy, 37
tendon,
   division, 160
   grafts, 160
   injuries to,
      knee extensor mechanism, 191
      finger, 160, 162
      thumb, 161
   repair, 160
   rupture,
      biceps, 69, 129
      extensor pollicis longus, 162
      finger extensors, 33, 162
      tendo-Achilles, 69
   sheath,
      giant cell tumour of, 70
      inflammation of,
         acute, 67
         chronic, 68
         rheumatoid, 33
         stenosing, 68
         subacute, 68
      transplants, 38, 39
tennis elbow, 133
tenosynovitis, see tendon sheath
test,
   finger extension, 134
   HLA antibody, 109
   latex agglutination, 35
   McMurray's, 189
   Mills, 134
   Ortolani's, 169
   patella compression, 12
   Rose–Waaler, 35
   Thomas' hip flexion, 9
   tourniquet, 30
   Trendelenberg's, 10
tetraplegia,
   anatomy, 97
   cord damage, 99
   definition, 99
   management, 112
thenar muscle paralysis, 28, 30
Thomas' hip flexion test, 9
Thomas' splint, 181
thoracic spine,

Scheuermann's disease, 101
scoliosis, 101
thoraco-lumbar spine,
   ankylosing spondylitis, 109
   fracture-dislocations, 111
thumb,
   anatomy, 155
   Bennett fracture-dislocation, 164
   examination, 13
   fractures, 164
   ligament strains, 165
   movements, 155
   muscles acting on, 156
   osteoarthrosis, carpo-metacarpal joint, 149
   trigger, 160
tibia,
   anterior tibial syndrome, 192
   congenital pseudarthrosis, 196
   fractures,
      condyle, 195
      malleolus, 205–7
      shaft, 197
      spine, 195
   osteotomy, 187
   tibial tubercle, avulsion of, 191
toenail,
   ingrowing, 206
   onychogryposis, 217
toes,
   arthroedoesis of, 215, 216
   claw, 215
   fractures, 218
   hammer, 214
Tom Smith's arthritis, 171
torticollis,
   infantile, 94
   scoliotic, 94
   spasmodic, 93
traction,
   definition, 17
   fixed, 181
   in immobilization of fractures, 17
   sliding, 181
   weight and pulley, 181
trapezium, excision in osteoarthrosis, 149
traumatic paraplegia,
   assessment, 99
   causes, 111
   level of injury, 111
   management, 112
   'root escape', 112
Trendelenberg's sign, 10, 170, 176
trigger finger, 69
trochanteric fractures, 178
tuberculosis,
   dactylitis, 46
   osteomyelitis, 44
   paraplegia in, 45
   of pelvis, 116
   spine, 45

Index 231

tumours,
  acoustic neuroma, 31
  aneurysmal bone cyst, 80
  arterio-venous aneurysm, 81
  brown, 61
  chondroma, 75
  chondrosarcoma, 76
  diaphyseal aclasia, 56
  dumbell tumour of spine, 32
  enchondroma,
    multiple, 57
    single, 75
  Ewing's, 77
  exotosis, 72
  fibroma
    of bone, 75
    of soft tissue, 81
  fibrosarcoma,
    endosteal, 75
    periosteal, 75
    of soft tissue, 81
  ganglion, 69
    of flexor tendon sheath, 160
    of wrist, 148
  giant cell tumour
    of bone, 77
    of tendon sheath, 70
  glomus, 81
  leiomyoma, 81
  leiomyosarcoma, 81
  leukaemia, 79
  metastasies in bone, 80
  multiple exostoses, 56
  multiple myelomatosis, 78
  myeloma, 78
  osteochondroma, 72
  osteoid osteoma, 79
  osteosarcoma,
    in Paget's disease, 74
    primary, 73
    secondary, 74
  osteotoma, 72
    cancellous, 72
    ivory, 72
    osteoid, 79
  parosteal sarcoma, 75
  periosteal fibrosarcoma, 75
  plasmacytoma, 78
  rhabdomyoma, 81
  rhabdomyosarcoma, 81
  synovioma,
    benign, 70
    malignant, 71
  tendon sheath, 69
tunnel syndromes,
  carpal, 30
  radial, 134
  tarsal, 31
  ulnar, 29

ulna,
  fractures,
    coronoid process, 139
    olecranon process, 138
    shaft, 143
    styloid process, 149
ulnar
  nerve,
    compression at wrist, 29
    innervation in, 156
    neuritis, 29
    paralysis, 27
    release, 29
    transposition, 29
  paradox, 28
urethra, damage to, in pelvic fractures, 119
uric acid levels, 83
urogenital tract, injuries, 119

valgus, definition, 3
varus, definition, 3
vertebra,
  anatomy,
    cervical, 97
    general, 91
  anomalies,
    congenital, 93, 105
    in mucopolysaccharide disease, 59
  injuries, *see* relevant region of spine
  ossification, 92
  osteochondritis, 101
verticle compression fracture of ankle, 207
villonodular synovitis, 86
Volkmann's ischaemic contracture, 140
von Recklinghausen's disease,
  of bone, 61
  of nerve, 31
Von Rosen's lines, 169

weight-relieving caliper, 18
Wormian bones, 55
wrist,
  anatomy, 146
  carpal tunnel syndrome, 30
  de Quervain's syndrome, 147
  examination, 9
  fractures,
    Barton's, 151
    Colles', 149
    lunate, 153
    radial styloid, 152
    scaphoid, 152
    Smith's, 150
  fracture-separation of lower radial epiphysis, 149
  ligament injuries, 149
  Madelung's deformity, 146
  movements, 9
  rheumatoid disease, 148
  tenosynovitis, 147